# FIGHT
# FATIGUE

*Six Simple Steps to Maximize Your Energy*

## MARY ANN BAUMAN M.D.

TATE PUBLISHING, LLC

"Fight Fatigue" by Mary Ann Bauman M.D.
Copyright © 2005 by Mary Ann Bauman M.D. All rights reserved.

Published in the United States of America
by Tate Publishing, LLC
127 East Trade Center Terrace
Mustang, OK 73064
(888) 361–9473

Book design copyright © 2005 by Tate Publishing, LLC.
All rights reserved.

Cover Photography: KENN BIRD/kennbird.com

No part of this publication may be reproduced, stored in a
retrieval system or transmitted in any way by any means,
electronic, mechanical, photocopy, recording or otherwise
without the prior permission of the author except as provided by USA copyright law.

This book is designed to provide accurate and authorita-
tive information with regard to the subject matter covered.
This information is given with the understanding that
neither the author nor Tate Publishing, LLC is engaged
in rendering legal, professional advice. Since the details of
your situation are fact dependent, you should additionally
seek the services of a competent professional.

ISBN: 1–5988618–7-5

*to Bart and Lauren*

# ACKNOWLEDGMENTS

The first time someone suggested that I write a book, I was caught off guard. It was September 1991, and I had just finished speaking to an audience of women at Integris Baptist Medical Center in Oklahoma City. The person who made that remark was Gary Good, who booked our national speakers. When I questioned him, he patiently repeated his statement and told me that he thought I had a lot to say. I had been recommending many of my techniques to my patients for years, but I was not sure that I could find the time to actually sit down and write. After all, I had a family, a practice, a home, and an active, fulfilling life. It was a daunting project to consider.

However, it was my sister Nancy who finally got me started. She had read of an author who forced himself to write for just one hour a day, every day, and suggested that I try that technique. It would not matter how much I wrote, but I had to sit there for the full hour. I compromised—one hour a day was just too much so I decided on one hour each week. Believe me, the first few weeks were torture! I'd write a paragraph and then delete it. Mostly, I'd watch the clock. But then, a surprising thing happened. After I made an outline and organized my thoughts, the words started to flow. One hour became two and then three and over the next 18 months, I wrote this book.

So much credit goes to Gary Good for planting the seed and to Nancy for getting me started and supporting me throughout the process.

You'll find I tell a lot of stories about my family, my friends, and my patients. That's because I've learned a great deal from all of them throughout the years. My parents, Bob and Bernadine Bauman, have a passion for learning. They believed in educating their daughters during an era when that was not the conventional wisdom, and my sisters and I are the beneficiaries of their foresight. They taught me the rewards that come from hard work, hard play, and always putting family first. My four siblings are all accomplished in their fields and dedicated to their families. Bob shows me unending determination, Therese, outstanding organizational skills, Michele, extreme patience, and Nancy, perceptive insight with humor. We have made the transition from childhood playmates to adult friends, and I am grateful for and to each one of them.

I must give heartfelt thanks to my sister, Michele. She is the busy mother of three beautiful daughters, holds a full time position at General Motors, is the right hand of my parents and yet found the time to edit the first draft of my manuscript. Believe me, she is a tough editor, and I love her for her efforts and support.

A special note of acknowledgment must also go to my dearest friend, Cathy Keating. She, too, reviewed the very early draft and her comments were invaluable—another picky editor! More importantly, her friendship is an anchor in my life. It is comforting to share our lives and families, and I am so appreciative of her love and support. We have a rich tapestry of memories, and we add new ones all the time.

Speaking of editors, Gary Bokelmann is a wonderful one. A talented writer in his own right, he is adept at making sure I don't fall into "doctor speak." We have collaborated a few times, and he always knows just how to tweak a phrase if it's not quite clear. Gary, someday we'll have to meet in person.

Stacy Baker, my editor at Tate Publishing, deserves my thanks for her meticulous attention to detail and her enthusiasm for this project. Kenn Bird, my neighbor and a phenomenal professional photographer, is responsible for the cover photo, and Sommer Buss, Creative Director, Tate Publishing, is to be credited for the cover design. I appreciate their talent and creativity.

Last, but certainly not least, I must thank my family. Tom and Dan, you taught me how blended families work. Thanks for hanging in with me when I didn't always do it well, for embracing your little sister and for making us truly a family. I love you both and am proud of the men you have become.

Lauren, what can I say? There is a reason you figure so prominently in many of my stories. As I've always told you—being your mom has been my best and most important job. I have learned from you and with you. I remember when you were just a little girl and you asked me if you were my best friend. You were disappointed when I told you honestly that you were just a little too young for that. Well, my daughter, you're not too young anymore. I cherish our times together and love watching as you mature and face life's challenges with intelligence and grace.

Finally, Bart, love of my life, I owe you my deepest gratitude. Together, we have weathered happy and sad times, been wonderfully successful and deeply disappointed. Through it all, we've made each other better. You have shown me what unconditional love looks and feels like. Life with you is the best!

MARY ANN **BAUMAN, MD**

# TABLE OF CONTENTS

# FOREWORD

I f you saw this classified ad in the newspaper, would you answer it?

If you fit the description above, and especially if you've found that no one can be "superwoman" forever, this book was written just for you.

Those who know me, particularly those who have known me throughout my lifetime, may wonder why I am writing the foreword to Dr. Bauman's book *Fight Fatigue: Six Simple Steps to Maximize your Energy*. I confess! I am fortunate to have enormous amounts of energy, but I haven't always been like

**Help Wanted**

**Job Description**
Hard-working woman who is superb at multitasking, personifies "Ms. Everything to Everybody," and is talented, loving, kind, understanding, smart, selfless, loyal, devoted while being "Johnnie-on-the-spot." Needs to have difficulty saying "no." Must be available 24/7.

**Titles**
Wife, mother, daughter, sister, friend, professional, volunteer—SIMULTANEOUSLY

**Salary**
Unavailable

**Benefits**
Rewards too many to mention

**Cost** Exhaustion!

**Applicants**: READ ON

the "Energizer Bunny." In fact, a few years ago my battery ran dry. I hit the "fatigue barrier" that lurks out there for all of us, whether we believe it or not. So I have a vested interest in helping the good doctor share her formula for helping others recharge their personal batteries. Yet there is more. Dr. Bauman—Mary Ann—is my dearest friend, as well as my personal physician. She is a second mother to my children, Carrie in particular, and she is a substitute grandmother to my precious, perfect grandchildren, Catie and Will. As mothers, women, and friends, we have spent a great deal of time traveling the road of friendship reenergizing our lives together.

For most of my life, I have been blessed with an over abundance of energy—energy that many wished they had and several of them certain that I attained by taking some *magic potion* every day. What in the world could I possibly know about fatigue? I was the child who never wanted to go to bed at night. I certainly wasn't tired, and I just might miss something. Additionally, I wiggled my way through school. As a child, this much energy can be perceived as a nuisance to teachers, and it can and did exhaust my parents at times.

As an adult, this enormous sum of energy came to be expected by me and envied by many. For me it was simply the norm, as I did not know any differently. But please do not misunderstand. I am not Wonder Woman. I, too, have suffered from bouts of exhaustion, which come from taking college finals, early motherhood filled with sleepless nights, and working while rearing a family. However, the difference for me was that I expected to be tired during those times as that just comes with the territory. Besides, I always bounced back easily.

Just imagine the personal consternation I felt when, over a relatively short period of time, my energy level collapsed, and it did so while my husband was Governor of Oklahoma. I, too, was in a very public role. Being a typical female, I suffered in silence. I did not want to disappoint or let anyone down. Plus, I certainly did not want to alarm anyone so I just kept going.

In the back of my mind, I worried that I could have some dreaded, life-threatening illness. I wondered if I should bother my doctor and friend, Mary Ann, with this or might this feeling of exhaustion just disappear after several good nights of sleep? My better judgment finally prevailed, and I made an appointment to see Mary Ann. For the first time ever, I was experiencing fatigue differently, and it was up close and personal. It wouldn't go away and I was devastated. I was alarmed, and I wanted a quick fix. If there was one, I knew that Mary Ann would prescribe it for me. After all, she always got me well.

Does this story sound all too familiar? Of course, the details of your journey might be different, but I suspect that you are reading this because the symptoms are the same. You, too, are tired of being tired! And you, too, don't know how to remedy the problem. The good news for me was that after determining there wasn't a thing wrong with me medically, what I suffered from was fixable. I hope that the same will be true for you. And, yes, there is a *magic potion* Mary Ann prescribed for me that can help you as well. You are holding it in your hand!

In the first chapter, you will discover how self-esteem is directly linked to energy or lack thereof. Reading *Woman—Pleasing Everyone but Herself,* I learned how important it is to "give myself permission" to "let go" of people's unkind behaviors in life. Believe me, in the world of politics people can fabricate the most outrageous stories and the ensuing emotion is always a downer! "If people knew better they would do better" is my mother's philosophy, which has helped me keep destructive comments at bay throughout my life. Since reading this chapter, I discovered that letting go of these behaviors comes with the bonus of being an energy booster as well! So basic. So easy. So very doable. And just one of the many tips yet to come.

My journey to reclaim my energy started with this same plan. To begin, just read this book. It is a fun read as Mary Ann is a master storyteller and her real life stories make it easy for each of us to identify. There are also stories that bring to light the feeling of "been there/done that" and of "misery loves company," which illustrate why we need to read on! Each story builds on the next, becoming a powerful motivation to get the show on the road. Of course, while reading this book, you will discover what your personal plan needs to be and how YOU must call it into action. I found that to be easy. The only difficulty is in making the commitment to move to action and then sticking with it. Only you can make that commitment, and it is something that you really must want to do. That is the difference in success or failure and whether you will experience this wonderful new-found surge of energy and all that accompanies it.

For me, once the commitment was genuinely made, everything else fell in place, and in time, Dr. Bauman's *magic potion* took effect. My energy soared again. My positive attitude returned. The "old" me was back once more—making lists, loving life, and being pleased with myself! And to think that it all started with a simple journey that ultimately gave me a new lease on life. What an amazing gift to my family, my friends, and yes, to myself!

This is why I wanted to be a part of Dr. Bauman's book—as I want you to experience the same success in reclaiming your energy and your life that I experienced, with her help and advice.

The prescription is here, and best of all, it puts the outcome squarely in your hands.

Now if Dr. Bauman can just find a way to convince me to give up Diet Cokes!

**Cathy Keating**

First Lady of Oklahoma 1995–2003

*Wife, mother, daughter, friend, professional, community volunteer, etc., etc., etc.*

# WHO AM I AND WHY DID I WRITE THIS BOOK?

*"Doctor, please help me! I barely have
enough energy to get through my day."*

**D**oes this sound familiar? It certainly does to me. I've heard this lament countless times over the past 25 years from female patients. And it's no wonder—all of us are busy juggling home, work, and family obligations.

Our lives are fast-paced and, we hope, satisfying. Yet the price we pay can cause us to overlook even the good things that happen every day.

After all, if we don't have energy, nothing is fun and even simple tasks can become a chore.

Fortunately, there is a way out. It is possible to generate the energy you need and deserve. However, it may require you to take a different approach than you have in the past. You can't just pop a pill or even vow to wait it out as you do when you have a cold. No, in order to begin truly enjoying life again, you may need to look beyond the physical reasons for fatigue and consider the emotional facets of your life as well. In short, what you need is to find your mind-body balance.

We have a tendency to think of energy as something physical—either something you have or you don't. We generally measure it in terms of the number of tasks we are able to perform, but that doesn't really give us an accurate or complete picture. Energy is also defined by your emotional state—your overall sense of well-being and the satisfaction you feel from the relationships in your life. These factors have as much impact on your energy levels as the physical demands on your time.

Now you may wonder why a medical doctor is writing about your emotional state and your relationships. Isn't that more suitable for someone trained in psychiatry or psychology rather than internal medicine? Why should you believe that an internist who focuses on mind-body balance has a plan that will improve your energy? Why am I not focusing on the diseases that cause fatigue?

These are certainly legitimate questions. As a primary care doctor, I have done the medical evaluation for fatigue on hundreds of women who are tired. Invariably, I am the first doctor that she will approach, and I always start with a thorough history and physical exam, blood tests, and x-rays to look for a medical reason for my patient's lack of energy.

I diligently search for a metabolic or physiologic abnormality that might explain the symptoms, and sometimes I do find the cause. For example, the thyroid activity may be low, the blood sugar level may be high, or the woman could be anemic. I look for signs of heart disease or depression because fatigue frequently goes hand-in-hand with these diagnoses. I always recommend that a tired patient undergo a detailed evaluation. Still, for the majority of my patients, the tests all come back normal. Now this is a good thing. After all, I don't want my patients to be sick. However, I am still left with a woman who is tired and who is looking to me for an answer. She wants to feel better. She wants to have the energy to satisfy her daily obligations and enjoy her life.

Ironically, it is often frustrating for the patient to be told that all is fine because she's still tired and doesn't know where to turn. It's also frustrating for doctors when we can't help our patients to feel better. It is this mutual dissatisfaction that led me to search for an approach that would help these women find their energy.

Although I am an internist, I have always been drawn to the mind and its immense influence over our well-being. In the 1980s, I served as the Internal Medicine liaison to the Department of Psychiatry at the University of South Dakota College of Medicine and took care of the medical needs of psychiatric patients. In that role, I was struck over and over again by how much physical health is influenced by emotional issues.

Some of this is not new. Throughout the years, there have been reports in the medical literature about dramatic cases where a patient might, for example, have a completely paralyzed arm or leg, yet there is absolutely nothing medically wrong with the limb. The physical symptoms are purely the result of a severe emotional trauma. There is even a name for this condition: it's called a conversion reaction because the patient converts emotional stress into physical symptoms.

There are clear links between emotional and physical health. I will outline scientific studies that dramatically illustrate just how much influence the mind has over the body. Then we will explore how a new approach, one that enables you to evaluate how and why you make your life choices, can generate a wellspring of energy that lets you take on the challenges of your everyday life with enthusiasm.

You will read about women not so different from yourself, women who have faced and won the energy battle, as well as women who are still struggling with it. Their stories will give you valuable insights, but you will also gain much more. After all, insight alone is not enough. My purpose is not simply to help you understand why you are tired, but also to help you to achieve balance and to tap into the energy that balance generates.

That's why a key component of this book is the step-by-step plan it outlines. The steps are designed to put you on the path to mind-body balance. If you are not ready to take action, to face up to your personal energy thieves, then this plan is not for you. It will require effort, of course, but more importantly, it will require a commitment to identify and implement a mind-body balance in your life.

I'm not offering a pill, a therapy, or even a diet. This is a six-step program that will increase your energy. It is designed to easily become a part of your daily life so that you can maintain your newfound vigor. Mind-body balance will become a habit.

At this point you may well ask, "How do I know it will work?" Another fair question. After all, I'm asking you to commit time—not only to read this book but also to make changes in your life—and time is a precious commodity these days.

The best reassurance I can provide is to tell you how my approach was developed.

As an internist, I have addressed the medical needs of both women and men in my primary care practice over two decades. As the Internal Medicine faculty member who worked with psychiatrists, I have observed firsthand the power of the mind. As an advocate for women's health issues, I have delivered hundreds of talks and participated in countless seminars with and about women. As a wife, mother, daughter, sister, friend, et al, I have searched for balance in my own life. I have heard women of all ages decry their lack of energy and have seen how this can rob a woman of joy as she goes about her life's activities. Did you know that fatigue is the most common reason that women go to the doctor? This is not true for men. I wondered why.

I began to explore the differences in how we approach our tasks, our relationships, and the challenges in our lives. I assessed my female patients and compared those who had energy with those who did not. I listened to countless women in my seminars commiserate about their frustrations, about the number of people they took care of, and about their exhaustion. It didn't seem to matter whether they worked outside of the home or not; they were tired. I looked at men—those in my practice and those in my life. In preparation for my talks, I read the medical literature, and slowly,

MARY ANN **BAUMAN, MD**

over the years, a realization occurred: The very same nurturing spirit that makes us such devoted moms and caretakers is also responsible for our energy crises. This was an eye-opener for me.

At the same time, the medical literature on the importance of the mind-body connection began to explode. Psychoneuroimmunology (the scientific term for the mind-body connection) became a legitimate and active field of research. I read the studies avidly, gave many talks on the subject, and became more and more convinced that this was not simply an interesting research phenomenon. The mind-body connection impacts our lives on a daily basis.

Armed with this new insight, I began to look at my patients' energy woes in a different light. I began to explore not just the demands on them but also how they interpreted those demands, how they felt about them, and why they continued to do things they didn't want to do for people they didn't like.

I also evaluated my own responses to my responsibilities and compared them with the responses of my husband. He's a very nurturing guy, but he does have that male chromosome! Slowly, after years of study and observation, I began to change my behavior. I began to pay attention to my personal mind-body connection and to turn that attention into positive action. I evaluated the relationships in my life in light of this new insight and set boundaries and made changes when I was unhappy. It wasn't always easy and I wasn't always right, but the rewards have been tremendous. Not only do I have a sense of well-being but my energy level has soared. I have the tools to juggle all of my responsibilities without losing sight of my own needs.

Because I have always taken the health and wellness of my patients very seriously and personally, I began to speak enthusiastically about the importance of these issues to their energy balance. I urged them to do their own mind-body evaluations as a prelude to making the changes that would allow them to increase their energy. Some listened, some didn't. Those who embraced the concept, who were willing to do the work, were rewarded.

Others, however, with the best of intentions simply did not have the energy for an in-depth analysis. Let's face it—if you are overwhelmed with daily demands, if you are tired from the moment you awaken in the morning until you close your eyes at night, you likely will not be inclined to spend much time analyzing why. It became clear that for this approach to be effective, I would have to develop a plan that was simple and, above all, not time-consuming.

It is this plan that you will see outlined in the chapters that follow. It is easy and designed to be implemented during your regular daily activities. It does require a commitment but one that is not onerous or excessive. The steps are designed to start you on the path, to convince you of the importance of the mind-body-spirit connection, and to give you the tools that you will need to maximize your energy. However, this plan will pay other dividends as well. Not only will you have more energy, you also will find that your relationships with your family, friends, and coworkers will improve. You will be able to focus on the tasks at hand without the extraneous concerns that wear you down.

Now if you happen to be a person who has lots of energy, you might think that this book is not for you. After all, you don't have a problem meeting all of the demands on your time. Right? Actually, you will find that if you follow the steps and make them a part of your daily routine, you will not only protect the energy you have today, you will increase the amount available tomorrow. This is essential because there are always those occasions when energy demands escalate, and it is important to have reserves to meet the additional challenges.

When I finally sat down to write, I began to consider the details. I knew what I wanted to say. I knew that the concepts would work, but I wasn't sure about the organization of the book—how many chapters, how should they be structured, and so forth. Luckily, as I was mulling these questions (actually, worrying, if the truth be told!) I had dinner with a group of friends. One of them asked me about my work, and as I described my ideas, she commented, "I hope you'll make it a small book." When I asked her why, she explained that she didn't have a lot of free time so she really enjoyed books that did not take forever to read.

That comment proved to be quite important to me. I decided to quit worrying about producing an epic and just take as much time as I needed to outline my plan. So think of this as the little, big ENERGY book.

A final note before you begin: What we will be talking about is attainable and will fit into the busiest of schedules. The energy building concepts in this book will lead to greater satisfaction with your life and can work for you as they have for me and for others. Remember, you are not the only one who will benefit from your newfound energy. Those you love and care for will appreciate the difference.

So come begin the journey with me. After all, what have you got to lose—except that tired, dragged-out feeling?

# CHAPTER 1

# WOMAN—PLEASING EVERYONE BUT HERSELF

You may wonder what self-esteem has to do with energy, but as we are about to discover, the two are intricately linked. Understanding self-esteem and understanding how we develop and nurture it are each important steps in your quest for more energy, both emotional and physical.

Self-esteem is a much-used, some would say abused, concept these days, but there is no denying its influence over our lives. It is how we judge our own "worthiness." It is the attitude each person has about herself or himself, and it does affect behavior. Be aware that many of the decisions you make in your daily life are influenced by your desire, conscious or unconscious, to feel good about yourself.

There are researchers who believe that a person's self-esteem is partly genetically determined, while others contend that it is highly influenced by one's environment, both familial and societal. However, regardless of the weight they give to genetics, virtually all experts agree that environment plays a major role in developing self-esteem. What is even more significant is that boys and girls—and later, men and women—develop self-esteem differently. Boys learn very early on that self-esteem comes from accomplishing tasks, while girls are conditioned to achieve self-esteem through relationships with other people. This is a generalization, of course, but the difference is significant, and it impacts both sexes throughout their lives.

Neither of these approaches is inherently "bad," but like so many things in life, each is something of a double-edged sword. For example, we've all heard stories of successful men who are so goal-oriented that they ignore the relationships in their lives. The downside of such a task-driven self-esteem model is clear: One can be a great provider of material goods and yet, sadly, lose the love of spouse and children.

But what are the drawbacks to the oppo-

MARY ANN **BAUMAN, MD**

site approach? What happens to those who are *too* relationship-oriented? Most women are wonderful nurturers. We care greatly about all of the people in our lives: family members, colleagues, subordinates, friends, and even just acquaintances. This makes us great wives, mothers, and friends, but there's a downside. We run the risk of becoming obsessive people-pleasers who constantly require the approval of others—at the risk of our own physical and mental well-being.

## The Burdens We Impose on Ourselves

Has this ever happened to you? There is someone you don't like and don't respect. To tell the truth, you think he or she has few redeeming qualities. Yet if that person doesn't think you're the "best thing since sliced bread," you become upset! You wonder what you did wrong, and it bothers you. What's worse, you keep searching for ways to win that person's approval and respect—*even though you will never feel that way about him or her.*

I know this happens because it has happened to me, and it is very unsatisfying, not to mention exhausting. I once had a colleague who was boorish, chauvinistic, and antagonistic. He did not treat me well. Does this sound like anyone you know? Nevertheless, I found myself constantly wondering what *I* had done to warrant his reaction.

Even more significantly, I kept asking myself what I could do to make him like and respect me. I thought if I would just work a little harder, he would see the light. It was only after I had tried over and over again to gain his approval that I finally stopped to evaluate the situation.

When I did that, I came to two conclusions. First, I had not behaved inappropriately; the problem really was his, not mine. And second, if I was completely objective, his approval was not even valuable to me!

It did take some time, but eventually the light went on in my head. I realized that it was *my* need for approval that kept me running in a race that I didn't really need or want to win. However, as simple and straightforward as this sounds, I must tell you that I wasted a lot of energy before I reached this "obvious" conclusion.

And that's the problem. If you take my initial reaction to this encounter and multiply it by the number of encounters with different individuals I have each day or week or month, you can begin to see just how tiring this approval-seeking response can be. That's what you need to realize. Identifying and understanding your reactions has practical consequences to your energy balance.

For you, this analysis process may involve your kids, people at church, your coworkers, or any of the myriad people who make up your life. You may find yourself being pulled in many different directions as you try to meet everyone's needs and expectations. You give equal weight to every request, and it becomes impossible to keep up.

Ultimately, however, even the good things, the activities you truly enjoy, become a hassle because you are tired. You never stop to think about why you feel compelled to say "yes" to a particular request when the practical part of you knows full well that you don't have the time. Heaven forbid that you say "no" just because you don't want to do it. That would be *selfish,* and we all know that being selfish is wrong.

Or is it? Certainly, there are inconsiderate people who put their personal needs above all others, but for the majority of women that is not the case. Our self-esteem antenna would never permit that. We just become exhausted instead.

These self-esteem cravings can be sneaky. If we constantly seek these "hits" to our self-esteem and never stop to realize why we need that approval, we can quickly deplete our energy reserves. Soon I will challenge you to begin the process of evaluating the relationships in your life. It is critical to your energy balance that you identify these self-esteem issues for yourself. Certainly, until you take this first step, you will not be able to change your behavior. And that's the key—identifying and changing those behaviors that suck the energy out of your life and result in unhappiness, discontent, and exhaustion.

## Fathers and Children

A study evaluating the interactions of parents with their young children found that fathers teach their sons and daughters differently (Frankel).

Picture this example because it illustrates so well how gender related differences develop. A little boy is putting together a puzzle. He reaches a point where he says, "Daddy this is too hard." Dad responds with words of encouragement such as, "Keep trying, Son, you can do it." The little boy does keep trying and eventually is successful.

Now think of this identical scenario with a young daughter instead. She reaches the same point, "Daddy, this is too hard." What do you think her father says? You guessed it! "Here, honey, let me help you." Therefore, while the little boy learns the importance of persistence and the satisfaction of accomplishing a task, the little girl learns to depend on her relationships with others for success.

A perfect illustration of this occurred in my own life. When our daughter was seven years old, I decided she needed a task to do during the summer. I wanted it to be something that would be her responsibility and which she could easily master so that she would experience a sense of accomplishment.

After much thought—you know how we

compulsive mothers are—I decided she would be responsible for weeding the flowerbed in front of our house. This bed is about 12 feet long by 3 feet wide. I dutifully divided it into six 2-foot segments (I told you I was compulsive!) and showed her just how to do the weeding. The entire task would take only five or ten minutes each day, and by the end of the week she would have weeded the whole bed.

Being a typical child, Lauren wanted no part of this. She did not want to do her simple chore, and she objected repeatedly and vociferously. Finally, she called me at work one day and told me again why she "couldn't," read that as "wouldn't," do this. In my best "this is it" voice, I told her to go outside and get started.

Predictably, she called her dad instead. When I got home from work, my daughter met me at the door and told me that Daddy had said he would help her. She then turned to me with a knowing smile and added, "But I know he'll do it!"

Now Lauren was always a precocious child, but she did not realize that the first thing I would do when her dad got home was tell him what our little darling had said. He and I had discussed these self-esteem issues involving fathers and daughters before, and his response was most interesting. He said that if our older sons had ever told him they couldn't weed at this age, he would not have hesitated to tell them to "Get outside and do it!" in no uncertain terms. However, in our daughter's case, he said somewhat plaintively, "But this . . . this is my little girl!"

To his credit, and in the interest of her self-esteem, he told her to get outside and do the weeding. But his initial instinct had been very different, and it was only because of his awareness that he altered his response.

It has been said that one of the major determinants of a young women's self-esteem is the nature of her relationship with her father at about age 6. So does this mean that if you didn't have a good relationship at that time you are forever doomed?

Absolutely not! When we understand our motivation, we can then take those behaviors that are healthy and nurture them, while we change those behaviors that are unhealthy and ultimately rob us of our sense of well-being. And make no mistake—you *can* change your behavior. It is hard work but incredibly rewarding. Understanding your motivation and where your impulses come from is the first step. Without that, you will never explore new ways to handle situations, and you will be doomed to continue the same frustrating and unsatisfying behaviors.

When I tell audiences about these studies of fathers and daughters, I always emphasize that we need to inform the men in our lives of these issues. That way, they can examine their responses to their daughters as my husband did with ours. Hopefully, as the future unfolds, young girls will be able to adopt a more balanced approach to self-esteem. Yet even if that doesn't happen, women do not have to give up precious energy constantly fighting these battles. We can choose another approach.

## Why a "Healthy Ego" Really Is Healthy

Any discussion of self-esteem and its effect on our energy would be incomplete without bringing up the subject of ego. During my talks, I always ask my audience members to call out what comes to mind when I say the word "ego." The responses are almost always the same: pride, selfishness, self-centered, and so forth. Invariably, someone will shout out "men" (not in a flattering way!) but only rarely will someone suggest a trait such as strength. The majority of responses define ego as a negative.

Well, I am here to tell you that ego is *not* bad. Ego defines our sense of self and is a valuable self-protective mechanism. It is our psyche's way of telling us that our plate is full. It is ego that allows us to say to our children, "I asked you if you wanted a ride and you said 'no,' so now I've made other plans." It is ego that lets us to say to our boss, "If I take on this new project, what should I drop?" It is ego that permits us to remind our husbands—and ourselves—that although we don't "have a job," we are working very hard.

Ego lets us make decisions that are in our best interests even if they don't fit society's conventional definition of success. I am reminded of a woman in my practice who came in for her annual physical one year and complained of being tired and quite stressed at work. She had recently accepted a new job that gave her a substantial raise in pay and status. Before she left, we talked a bit about the stressors she faced, and I did not hear from her again until she came in for her next exam a year later. At that time, she was feeling great. She had changed jobs and was extremely happy.

In the course of our conversation, I asked if her new job was financially as rewarding as the one she had left. Her answer was an emphatic "No!" She had taken a substantial cut in pay as well as status, but told me that it was absolutely worth it. She was enjoying herself, felt better, and had more time to exercise and take care of herself. She was back to her usual energetic state. I was impressed and told her so. It takes ego strength to make a decision that you know is right for you, but which might disappoint others or give the impression that you have failed.

If you don't pay attention to your ego, you will not feel well. You will be tired or your PMS will be out of control or you won't be able to sleep or you'll want to sleep all of the time or you'll be constipated or you'll have diarrhea or you'll have a headache or any of a variety of other uncomfortable symptoms. The bottom line: You will not feel well. You'll go to your doctor and your doctor will run tests, prescribe medications that may or may not work, and still you won't feel well.

Believe me when I say that I have seen this scenario over and over in my practice. Without ego, your self-esteem is challenged every time someone even hints at disapproval, whether he or she is family, friend, colleague, or acquaintance. With your self-esteem constantly at risk, you will find it impossible to establish reasonable boundaries as to what is expected of you. Life without boundaries is a chore; it is exhausting and it is unsatisfying.

Let me illustrate by telling you about a young woman in my practice. She was in her mid-30s, and she was distraught, depressed, exhausted, and angry. Her daughter was a typical teenager, her son needed chauffeuring all of the time, she could not find enough hours in the day to get everything done, and her husband didn't seem to understand her frustration, especially since she did not work outside of the home. To top it all off, her parents were coming for a visit and were going to stay at her house.

Although she loved her parents dearly, she was already anticipating her mother's disapproval because she was not a "perfect" housekeeper. She dreaded the extra work at mealtimes and the intrusion into her already busy household. When I suggested that she might have her parents stay at a hotel, she immediately and emphatically rejected the idea—not because they couldn't afford it, but because they would think her a "bad" daughter. Her self-esteem was caught up in her mother's approval, and it kept her from recognizing her own limits. (If we are honest, most all of us want our mothers' approval.) She did not have the ego strength to consider, let alone set, appropriate boundaries.

Eventually with the help of a talented counselor, she was able to analyze her behavior. With much trepidation, she broached the subject of a hotel to her mom. To her surprise, both parents readily agreed and they had a wonderful visit. She had more time and energy, and as a bonus, her young children enjoyed the hotel pool with their grandparents. In fact, it worked out so well that this has become their regular routine. Yet it was not easy for her to set up this very reasonable boundary because these self-esteem issues are powerful. Realize that a lack of ego often causes or exacerbates physical exhaustion.

That brings up another question: Did her mother really disapprove of her housekeeping in the first place? Or was that simply an assumption the daughter had made while she was wearing her self-esteem blinders? Sometimes we assume negative reactions that may never materialize, and if

MARY ANN **BAUMAN, MD**

we aren't careful, we will make decisions based on these erroneous assumptions.

Women are intuitive, and we generally do a good job of anticipating the needs of those around us. Nevertheless, we must recognize when we are in our "people-pleaser" mode. The need for approval takes over, our judgment becomes clouded, and we often make choices that threaten our energy balance.

Here's another example from my own experience: I am a runner, and I am religious about running four times each week. Shortly after we moved to Oklahoma, I took a break from the never-ending task of unpacking boxes and started stretching in preparation for my run. My husband walked into the room and asked if I was going to run. A few minutes later my daughter asked the same question. Neither said anything else, but I immediately felt defensive and thought about staying home instead.

Why? Because I interpreted the question as a sign of disapproval. When I objectively analyzed what they had said, there was nothing in either the content or tone that indicated any negativity. But just the same, I seriously considered changing my plans based on their *presumed* disapproval.

Although I was initially uncomfortable, I did complete my run that day and nothing further was said, either that day or the subsequent times I went out. In fact, my family often didn't even seem to notice when I was gone. That taught me a great lesson: My self-esteem antennae were so hypersensitive that I was ready to make a decision based on a false assumption about an innocent question. Indeed, that reaction threatened to keep me from making a very healthy decision.

## A New Approach to Energy and Self-Esteem

As you can see, self-esteem issues creep in even when they aren't invited. What's more, they *do* influence the choices you make and the energy balance you maintain. That's why it is critical for you to examine the day-to-day encounters in your life as you seek to restore or, in some cases, establish your mind-body balance.

That brings us to the first step of the new approach I promised you. This process consists of two main phases. First, you analyze the relationships in your life, and second, you take action. What I am proposing is not difficult and won't take long, but if it is going to work you must do it every day. Like so many things in life, the more effort you give, the more you will get in return.

Now before you close this book and complain, "I don't have time to do the rest of the things in my life so how can I add anything else?" Stop a moment. Take a deep breath and read on because the first step is quite simple and takes very little time.

## STEP 1: IDENTIFY

*At some time during your day, think about one encounter you had during the previous 24 hours. It may have involved a family member, friend, colleague, boss, or just someone at the grocery store. Now decide if that interaction made you happy or sad, satisfied or resentful, comfortable or uneasy.*

These are just examples, of course. You have a whole range of reactions from which to choose. As the days go by, try to recall a mix of both positive and negative experiences. That's all you have to do, just recall one encounter. However, you must do it every day. The best time for me is when I'm driving to or from work, but it really can be anytime—before you get out of bed, just after you get home, during your shower, or while you relax with a cup of coffee. Pick a time that works for you.

Be careful not to overanalyze the encounter, because at this point you will have a tendency to find fault with your reactions. You'll be tempted to berate yourself about what you should have said or could have done to "fix" the situation. That's not what this process is about.

That's also why it is critical that you choose

situations where the outcome was positive and you felt good about it, as well as those that didn't go so well. It is human nature to dwell on those situations that make you uncomfortable and to dismiss those that are satisfying. Guard against this mistake. There are many times during each day that you do things well. Now is the time to remember them because you are building a portfolio of "retrospective" reactions.

Eventually you will use this portfolio to learn how to change your behavior, but in this step all you do is identify your reaction to the situation and then let it go. You're finished for the day. Do this daily until it becomes a regular part of your life. Don't make the mistake of being so anxious to tackle your self-esteem issues that you try to shortcut the process. I am not proposing a quick fix. If you are going to achieve the results you desire, this step must be incorporated into your life. It must become a habit, and the only way that that will happen is by repetition. So keep at it.

While you work on identifying your reactions, let's move on to the fascinating topic of mind-body medicine. It's an interesting field with important implications to your energy and is a perfect introduction to the second step.

MARY ANN **BAUMAN, MD**

# CHAPTER 2

# POSITIVE THINKING
# PAYS BIG DIVIDENDS

I am absolutely convinced of the influence that the mind-body connection has on one's energy level. But *my* conviction is not enough. *You* must be convinced of the relevance to *your* life and *your* energy level. It is not enough to say, "Oh, that's interesting." Intellectual curiosity will not spur you to change behavior and—make no mistake—it will take a change in behavior to restore your energy balance. It will take action. Therefore, in this chapter, I will outline the evidence of the mind-body connection. My goal is to make this connection as relevant to your daily activities as it is to mine.

This whole concept has become an integral part of my practice of medicine as well as my personal life. I have found that I cannot properly evaluate a patient's symptoms without also inquiring about the person's stressors, relationships, and emotional health. These pieces of information affect not only the symptoms but also the disease states themselves.

I want you to be able to visualize this influence in your own life. As you read about the research and the examples that follow, challenge yourself to find instances from your own experience that might illustrate these concepts. I know you've had such experiences. It is merely a matter of remembering and thinking about the incidents from the perspective of the mind-body connection.

## Some Brief—but Necessary— Scientific Background

The subject of mind-body medicine is officially designated, "psychoneuroimmunology." I know that to the nonmedical person, it often seems that we go out of our way to choose the most convoluted, incomprehensible names we can find, but this one does make sense when you break it down: "Psycho" refers to the brain, "neuro" to the nervous system, and "immunology" to the immune system. Basically, input from the brain is transmitted to the body via the nerves, and the immune system acts as the controller of the resulting bodily processes. Thus psychoneuroimmunology describes the mind-body connection.

Norman Cousins is considered by many to be the father of psychoneuroimmunology. (Trust me, if you say it often enough, it begins to roll off your tongue quite easily!) You may have heard his story. He was the longtime editor of the *Saturday Review* who suffered from a disease that caused him significant and frequent pain. He noticed, however, that after he watched a funny movie—he liked Groucho Marx—he would experience several hours of blissfully pain-free sleep. He discussed this observation with his doctor, who took him seriously and did some rudimentary testing. Mr. Cousins chronicled his journey in a book called *Anatomy of an Illness as Perceived by the Patient: Reflections on Healing and Regeneration* (Cousins), and thus brought recognition to this emerging field of medicine.

Many studies were done in the 1980s. In one of these, young, healthy medical personnel were divided into two groups. The first group relaxed during quiet time, while the second group watched a comedian on video. At various intervals before, during, and after the session, blood was drawn from each participant to measure certain active substances such as cortisone, growth hormone, and epinephrine.

The results showed different levels of the hormones in the two groups. This was quite a significant finding because it showed that laughter did induce a different hormone reaction, and that the difference could be measured. Now it is important to realize that, although some of the substances measured are critical to our immune system response, this study indicated nothing about cause and effect. By that I mean that it was not designed to determine if the subject's health was improved by the laughter. It simply indicated that there was a definite and measurable response to the laughter. This study was one of the first to document hormonal responses to emotional reactions (Berk).

Other researchers found immune system responses were different depending on the subject's emotional state. In a study done on college students, it was found that those who were most stressed had decreased levels of IgA, a protein produced by the immune system (Jemmott). This protein is found in the nose and is thought to help the body fight colds.

The cynic may say, "So what? Mom always said that you get more colds when you are run down." Yes, moms are very wise, but these findings were important because they, once again, showed *measurable* changes in the immune system's response to an individual's *emotional* state. Again remember, this study did not show cause and effect; that is, they did not find that these students had more colds. That was not the goal. They *did* document lower levels of the protective protein and thus added to an increasing body of evidence to support the hypothesis that our emotional state does affect our physical well-being. Furthermore, and perhaps more important, studies like these suggest that the mechanism through which this mind-body connection functions involves the immune system.

## Your Mysterious Immune System

Have you ever just known that you were going to get sick? You've been burning the candle at both ends, pushing yourself too hard, and sure enough, you get a sore throat, your nose starts to run, and you get those familiar uncomfortable body aches that tell you that you're coming down with a cold. Then after a few days of misery, miraculously, you begin to feel better. The nose unclogs, the aches disappear, and you feel human again. This is your immune system at work. It revs up at the first sign of the virus and produces all kinds of infection-fighting cells that come to your rescue. That's "what" it does. The "how" has been more difficult to figure out.

When I was in medical school in the 1970s, we knew very little about this incredibly versatile system. In fact, it was referred to as a "black box," which means that we did not actually understand how it worked. We knew that when the body was faced with certain potentially injurious situations—exposure to bacteria, for example—the immune system processed this threat. If we were lucky, it produced an antibody or some other response that would protect or heal. We knew this, but we did not fully understand what happened inside that "black box" to produce the desired response.

Today, fortunately or unfortunately, we have a better understanding of how this system works. I say fortunately or unfortunately because our knowledge and understanding of the immune system grew by leaps and bounds beginning in the mid 1980s, continuing throughout the 1990s and into the present because of one devastating condition—AIDS. This horrible disease does not respect age, gender, sexual orientation, education, or socioeconomic level. It is an equal opportunity killer caused by the Human Immunodeficiency Virus (HIV) that systematically dismantles the immune system and renders it nonfunctional.

AIDS was first identified in the United States in the early 1980s and researchers began to dissect this disease in an effort to find a cure. As they studied the step-by-step failure of the body when infected with the virus, they were able to open the "black box" and began to figure out just how the immune system worked its magic. This was undeniably valuable information, but it has come at a tremendous price in lost human lives.

The explosion of knowledge acquired

because of this disease is the reason that I bristle when I hear people decry the amount of money spent on AIDS research. We have all benefited from this new knowledge about the immune system because it's not just about infections. For example, cancer is also an immune system disease. Why do I say that? Cells normally quit growing when they touch another cell. This is one of our body's mechanisms designed to keep things in check. However, in some types of cancer, cells lose that ability to recognize that it's time to stop expanding and reproducing. They keep dividing and growing and eventually form a mass—in this case, a cancerous tumor.

Now this is a very simplistic illustration of very complex functions, but I cite it so that you'll realize just how far reaching the immune system's influence is. Something happens to that cell's immune system response that causes it to lose this inborn protection. Also, no matter how careful you are, your body is exposed to carcinogens (cancer producing substances) all the time. You breathe them, touch them, eat them, and who knows what else with them! Yet your immune system delivers you from these threats again and again. It is truly a protector of your well-being. That's why it is so important that you do everything in your power to assist the process.

Heart disease can also be seen through this immune system filter. Do you know that atherosclerosis or hardening of the arteries begins at a young age, often in the teens or early twenties, and progresses through the years if you don't adopt a healthy lifestyle? It is not a disease that suddenly appears when you hit fifty. Heart disease is like the actor who becomes a star "overnight"—after twenty years of hard work.

This was quite apparent when autopsies were performed in the 1960s on Vietnam War casualties. Examiners found the beginnings of atherosclerosis in these young men who were, sadly, only in their late teens or early twenties. When the disease is allowed to progress unchecked throughout the decades, a point is finally reached when blood vessels become blocked or tiny pieces of atherosclerotic plaque break off, leading to a heart attack or stroke.

This then triggers an immune system response. Hormones are released and different cells travel to the site of injury and begin pouring out their contents. The process involves a very complex interaction of bodily reactions, all of which are orchestrated by the immune system. As our understanding grows, many new medicines are designed to interact with this immune system response in an effort to limit damage to and promote healing of the heart.

## The Power of Emotion—Can You Die of a Broken Heart?

There are a number of studies that have examined the subject of grief and our response to it. These, too, point to the importance of the mind-body connection. For example, it has been documented that in long-term marriages, after one's spouse dies, there is a statistically increased incidence of death of the surviving spouse within the first several years (Martikainen).

There are many theories as to why this occurs, with loneliness, loss of companionship, and loss of the will to live often being cited. I have my own personal opinion and it involves the immune system. I believe that during times of abject grief, something happens so that the immune system does not function at peak levels. Consequently, it does not perform its normal "surveillance" as well as usual, making the person more susceptible to a variety of illnesses, some serious and some not. Let me relate several experiences from my own life that will illustrate this concept.

My father-in-law died quite suddenly of a heart attack. My husband's parents had been married for over 50 years and retired to Florida eight years before his death. They had lived in Baltimore their entire lives, and I must confess that we were a bit skeptical when they announced that they were picking up and moving to Florida to enjoy their retirement. But that is precisely what they did.

They sold their old furniture, bought a lovely home, furnished it in tropical style, and proceeded to live life to the fullest. They joined clubs, were active in church, and enjoyed the beach frequently. It was always a treat to visit them; it was as though they had a new lease on life. So you can imagine just how overwhelming his loss was to my mother-in-law and to all of us. He was such a lovely man!

Margaret, my mother-in-law, went through a period of horrible grief. You could just feel her pain. I spoke with her every evening for nine months during this devastating time. Then gradually, she got a bit better. She emerged from the depths and resumed her life. She rekindled her interest in her clubs and started socializing again. She even made some wonderful lifestyle changes; she began exercising and quit smoking. That was amazing to me. She had been a lifetime smoker, and I never thought she'd quit, but she did.

She came for a Mother's Day visit about a year and a half after my father-in-law's death, and we had a wonderful time. We shopped, chatted over coffee, and even exercised together. She looked and felt wonderful. But then, three months later, she went in for her routine physical exam and a chest x-ray showed a shadow, which turned out to be a lung cancer. She elected not to take chemotherapy and moved in with us for the last six months of her life. We consulted Hospice, a truly wonderful service, and she died peacefully in our home, two years and three months after her husband's death.

Here was a woman who had smoked all her life, yet she didn't develop lung cancer until after her husband's death. Now the appropriate explanation may be that she was a lung cancer just waiting to happen. Yet in my heart of hearts, I believe that it was during that time of terrible grief that her immune system failed her, allowing those carcinogens to initiate the malignant transformation. The mind-body connection is a powerful force!

My daughter also had a most interesting reaction to her grandparents' deaths. She was seven at the time her grandfather died. Even though we lived in different states, they were always close. They spoke frequently over the telephone and sent tapes back and forth telling each other about the happenings in their lives. He was an avid Florida gardener and would always greet her with a cheery "Hi-biscus!"

We visited them that summer and the two of them had a wonderful time together spending hours at the beach riding the waves and exploring for sand crabs. Then early one Sunday morning in September, we received the phone call that everyone dreads. It was my mother-in-law calling to tell us he was gone, just like that. My father-in-law chose to be cremated so, although we had a memorial service, Lauren never saw him again. She once remarked to me in those first days that she never got to say goodbye, and his death was harder because of it.

Now for the mind-body angle: During the months following his funeral, Lauren repeatedly was sick with colds and sinus infections. I mean frequently, every few weeks or so. We'd just get over one and another would begin. It was very frustrating—so much so that in February of the next year I took her to the pediatrician. Now you have to understand I was not one to take her to the doctor very often, except for routine exams and shots. In fact, Lauren and my husband have always contended that they have to be "knocking on death's door" before I'll decide we need intervention. But in this case, I was becoming concerned that maybe something else was going on. The pediatrician heard my account, examined her, and said, "Of course she's getting sick. Her heart is broken."

She then explained that the average time of grieving for a child of this age was eight months. If her illnesses continued after that time, we should consider counseling to help her deal with the loss. Amazingly, after that eighth month she went back to her usual state of good health. Her spirit recuperated and her body did as well.

When her grandmother died, however, the situation was quite different. We had two rooms set up on the second floor of our home for my mother-in-law. She had a bedroom and a sitting room just down the hall from Lauren's room. They spent a great deal of time together during those six months. Early on, when Margaret could still get up and down the stairs, they would have breakfast together before school. When Lauren returned home, they would spend the late afternoon together talking and laughing. Lauren is a great aficionado of French. I think this comes from her grandmother, a French teacher, who during those times together transferred her love of the language and interest in the culture to her granddaughter.

Eventually Margaret required oxygen and became weaker and weaker. Lauren still recalls the sound of the oxygen concentrator making its swishing sound day in and day out. In fact, at one point she said with the honesty of a child, "Mom, I'm so tired of that sound all the time." Margaret, too, was growing weary and had reached the point when she prayed fervently for the end. When it did come, it was a peaceful and in the words of my husband, "an awesome experience." We spoke that afternoon of the love we all felt. She spent time with each one of us, and we each had the opportunity to say everything we wanted to say. She died that night.

The grief was sharp. Even when death is expected, you are never quite ready for the finality of it. She, too, chose to be cremated, and we had a lovely memorial service in Florida with family and friends. But here's what was most interesting: Lauren did not experience an upsurge in illness after her grandmother's death. I was expecting it, after what occurred two years earlier, but it just did not happen. She was very sad for a couple of weeks, but after that just seemed to have happy memories of her grandmother. She remarked often about how much she had enjoyed their time together and that she missed her, but her grief was definitely not as long lasting as when her grandfather died so abruptly.

I thought quite a bit about Lauren's different reactions over that first year and realized what a dramatic statement this experience made about the power of the mind-body connection. Lauren did her grieving, as did my husband and I, during those months before Margaret died. At the time of her actual death, we were all ready for it to be over, including Margaret herself. Therefore, the post-death grieving process was much shortened and Lauren did not have to spend the next months manifesting that grief with physical illness. Her heart "mended" much more quickly.

It is always interesting and, in a way, comforting for me to become aware of events in my own experience that illustrate the importance of keeping the mind healthy so that the body can be well. As a woman, I have to pay attention to these influences to help safeguard myself and those I love.

MARY ANN **BAUMAN, MD**

As a doctor, I have to be equally aware because my patients' health may very well be affected by events such as the ones I've described with my family.

In fact, I am so certain of the role that grief plays that I tell patients who have lost their spouses that they can expect not to feel well over the ensuing months. I tell them that I will watch them carefully, test when indicated, and reassure when appropriate. I encourage them to do only those things that are necessary during the first grief-stricken weeks to give themselves a chance to begin the healing process. I encourage them to rely on support systems, but to understand that one cannot rush the process. And I hope and pray that they will emerge from the experience healthy.

## A Matter of Attitude

One of my favorite studies about the mind-body connection reminds us in a very graphic way of the old saying about the glass being half empty or half full. You know the one I'm talking about—pessimists will see a glass as half empty while optimists see it as half full. It's all in your perspective because either way you have the same amount of liquid. Who would have thought, however, that this same idea could influence your health?

This wonderful study was begun in the 1940s with World War II veterans who were graduates of Harvard. They were interviewed about their war experiences and then followed over the next 35 years. Every 5 years, their personal physicians examined them and sent in a report. All of the men had similar wartime recollections, but their reactions to those events varied, as you might expect. What was so interesting and important was that those who had the most negative reactions to their experiences had a greater incidence of diseases between the ages of 40 and 60. The increase was statistically significant, which means there was more illness than could be explained simply by chance alone. After age 60, there were still more diseases recorded in this group, but the differences did not reach the level that was considered to be statistically significant (Peterson).

Think about this, and you'll begin to understand how very exciting these results were. Well before we could measure any of the hormones and active substances that were described in experiments years later—well before we understood much about the immune system at all—we had compelling information that suggested, rather dramatically, that attitude and emotional reaction could affect physical health. This was and is important.

Now the above study looked at the effect of pessimistic reactions, but is the opposite true? Does optimism affect your health in a positive way? Another study sought to evaluate this very question. In this case, researchers examined the relationship between an optimistic attitude and the incidence of heart disease in over 1300 veterans. They followed these patients for an average of 10 years and did, in fact, find less coronary artery disease, fewer heart attacks, and fewer deaths from heart attacks in the optimistic group (Kubzan-sky). Think about it; if you accept these results, it means that you accept that *you* have some control over what happens to your health.

Please understand, I do not mean to imply that if you suffer from a disease, it's because you have a bad attitude—obviously that's not true. But I do think it is important to look at your reactions, to learn from the events that happen in your life, and to try to see the positive whenever possible. We all know people who have been through extraordinarily painful situations. Yet after the initial shock and grieving period, they are able to return to a cheerful and upbeat attitude. We also know those who have been through lesser traumas who never seem to recover. I am suggesting that you do have some control over your reactions, and these studies suggest that the more positive you are, the better your chances of good health.

Now if you are one of those people whose natural tendency is to see the glass as half empty, finding the positive may sound like an impossible task. Don't despair! You can do it: Begin today to notice something good in your life. Put a Post-It note on your bathroom mirror or your desk at work that reminds you to "accentuate the positive!" It won't happen overnight, but with time and vigilance, you will see a change. We are often so caught up in the challenges we face that we ignore the many simple pleasant encounters that occur every day. Become aware of the small things. Recognize the beautiful sunshine during your morning drive to work rather than concentrating on the stressors you will face when you get there. Notice when someone smiles at you or your child gives you a quick hug. Eventually you'll find that if you concentrate on finding the positives every day, it will become second nature and you will do it automatically.

I try to do this in my own life. For example, spring is my favorite season because I am a summer person, and during springtime I know summer is not far behind. But spring is also a busy time of year, and if I am not vigilant, it can be gone before I've even thought about it. Therefore, I make it a point to notice each and every spring day. I started this several years ago, and now I find I never miss the enjoyment of this renewal season. Noticing spring has become a habit for me.

Find those positives in your life, even if they are not readily apparent, and you will discover a more optimistic you. Who knows, just as the studies of veterans suggested, it might lead to better health and perhaps even a better quality of life. My mom and dad are perfect examples. They have always believed that you can accomplish your goals as long as you are willing to do the work. They instilled these values in their children and taught us not to whine about circumstances but to strive to make them better.

Both of them have always admired those in the medical profession and that may be part of the reason why several of us chose to become doctors. I remember my father telling me that medicine would always be a noble calling, and that no matter what the technological advances, people would always need doctors. So far, even with the challenges in medicine these days, his words ring true. My parents have maintained an active life-style into their 80s, and I joke with them that they have a more active social life than we do.

You can then imagine our devastation when my dad suffered a severe stroke on Valentine's Day several years ago. He had had a bad cold and passed out while making coffee that morning. Initially, I thought this might have simply been cough-syncope, which means one faints during a violent coughing spell. It is not serious, but unfortunately, that was not his diagnosis. A CT scan showed a bleed into the brain. There are two basic types of strokes: ischemic, which is the most common, and hemorrhagic. In an ischemic stroke, blood flow to a particular area of the brain is blocked causing that part to sustain injury. In a hemorrhagic stroke, there is bleeding into the brain tissue itself and that causes the damage. Hemorrhagic strokes have a high risk of death in the first couple of days, and as you would expect we were all terribly frightened.

My dad did survive but was left with a total right-sided paralysis and an inability to speak. It was so frustrating for him not to be able to communicate his needs and for all of us to be unable to understand and help. After ten days in the hospital, he was transferred to a rehab facility to begin his journey to recovery. This is where my parents' optimism and commitment to hard work really paid off. The nurses commented that many patients were angry and unpleasant to the staff, but my dad always greeted them with a smile. My mom spent every moment at his side, from the time he got up in the morning until he went to bed at night. My sisters who lived in town were there virtually every day and those of us who lived out of state made the trip every 1–2 weeks. It was a difficult time.

Dad spent almost three months in rehab, and through incredibly hard work and with the help of dedicated therapists, he regained his function. It was amazing to watch. Now he is able to drive, and my parents have resumed their fulfilling, busy lifestyle. The point of this example is that my mom and dad had decades of optimism to fall back on when they needed it. Clearly they were frightened, as were we all, but they did not give up and had the reserves to meet the challenges they faced. This is why cultivating an optimistic attitude is important—you never know when it could be critical to your survival.

There is another study involving IgA that points out that your expectations can affect your immune system response. IgA is the immune system protein that we discussed earlier in the chapter. Undergraduate college students were divided into three groups. The first watched a film about IgA and listened to relaxing music. The second just listened to the music, and the third did neither. Researchers then measured each person's IgA level. Those in both music groups had higher levels of IgA, but the group that had watched the film had the highest levels (Rider). Thus their expectations affected their results.

In this same vein, a study was done on patients with upper respiratory infections who were coughing. If you've ever had a cold with a bad cough, you know that you often can't suppress that cough even when you try. The patients were told that the purpose of the study was to determine if vitamin E was helpful for coughs. Half of the subjects were given no medication and the other half of the group each took a vitamin E tablet. The researchers then recorded both the number of coughs and the length of time that the person could voluntarily suppress the cough over the next 15 minutes. Now understand that vitamin E, in reality, has no physiologic effect on cough and isn't even absorbed into the body for 2–4 hours after ingestion. So basically, neither group was given anything that would medically affect coughing.

Nevertheless, the vitamin E group had a 50% decrease in cough frequency and a significant increase in the amount of time that they could suppress a cough when compared with the other group (Lee). What do these examples tell you about the level of control you can exert over your body's reactions? Scientists are convinced of this effect, and that's why the best studies are blinded, which means that neither the subject nor the researcher knows which subject gets which treatment.

Dr. Stewart Wolf did a dramatic study about expectations back in 1950. Pregnant women who were experiencing morning sickness were told that they would be given medicine that would cure their nausea and vomiting (Wolf). You can be sure that this study was done a long time ago because no researcher today would take such risks with someone who is pregnant! Subjects were asked to swallow small balloons designed to measure contractions in the stomach. Then they were given ipecac, a medication that actually induces vomiting. It is used today in cases of poisoning when we want to clear the stomach out. Can you guess what happened? Their nausea and vomiting disappeared, and in one case, the stomach contractions actually returned to normal. Thus their *expectations* reversed the pharmacological action of the drug. Powerful reactions; powerful effects.

## Tuning in to the Mind-Body Connection

Throughout the years, I have met a number of patients who are very much in tune with their mind-body connection, and I have been amazed and humbled on more than one occasion. I remember a woman who came in and said, "Dr. Bauman, there is something wrong with my hormones. I have lost my serenity, and I've examined the other aspects of my life, and there is nothing going on that would account for this."

She had several other symptoms, which also pointed to the need for an adjustment in her hormone medications, but I've always remembered how clearly she approached this issue. Rather than starting, as patients often do, with a request for a medication to "fix" a problem, she did her own internal survey to determine her mind-body state. Only after she was convinced that that was in order did she look to medication.

I think this is a very healthy approach and indicates how you can practically and effectively use this connection in your daily life. But it will only work if you are in touch with the influences in your life and are able to do the assessment as my patient did. In order to do that you must first believe in the power of the mind-body connection. Now I hope the information I've already presented has helped you to do that. However, if you are still not convinced, listen to the following true account.

This patient shocked all of her doctors, me included, with her awareness and her extraordinary faith.

She was in her early forties and had been my patient for a number of years. She came in to see me late in August for her annual physical, and I noted that her left nipple was inverted. This means that instead of the nipple pointing out, it pointed in, similar to what you might see with the belly button. This can be normal, or it can mean that the nipple is being pulled in by a tumor in the breast. The usual question we ask is, "Is this new or has it always been this way?" If it has not changed over the years, then we do not worry. If it has, then we need to do further evaluation to be certain the patient does not have a breast cancer.

She told me that it had always been that way, and indeed, when I looked at my notes from previous years, I had recorded that the nipple was inverted. She had had a mammogram the year before and all had been fine then. Nevertheless, I did recommend another mammogram. She said she did not think she needed one this year but would agree to one the following year. She did not like to take medications or do a great deal of testing.

I did not hear from her again until several months later when I received a mammogram report that indicated a large mass, very suspicious for cancer in the left breast. I called her immediately to talk about it and asked her why she had had the test done, since she had decided against it earlier.

Her answer was profound in its simplicity. She said she knew something was not right with her body so she decided to check it out. We then spoke about the likelihood that this was cancer, and she calmly told me that she understood and agreed to begin the diagnostic process.

Here was a woman so in touch with her mind-body connection that she was able to decide on her own to have the mammogram done, even though earlier she had declined it. She had precisely and accurately pinpointed the problem. I asked her if the breast had changed, thinking that maybe she had felt a lump or some other abnormality that concerned her, but she said "no." I reminded her of our conversation about the inverted nipple. She remembered it and assured me that she and her husband had discussed this aspect as well, but both agreed that the breast was no different. She had just decided that since she didn't feel quite right, she needed to have the mammogram done.

She remained remarkably calm, accepting of the likely diagnosis of breast cancer, and was very optimistic. That in and of itself was noteworthy, but over the next year her story would become even more unusual.

Because the tumor was large and she was premenopausal (still having periods), chemotherapy was recommended to shrink the cancer before surgery. She began the treatments, but after a few months she developed a new lump that was found to be a new cancer. This was most unusual and, frankly, not a good sign. It meant that we were dealing with a very aggressive cancer. In other words, not only did it not get smaller with our treatment, another cancer actually formed even in the presence of the treatment drugs. This was very worrisome.

The oncologist spoke with the patient and her husband about a stem cell transplant that was being done at the time for aggressive breast cancer in the hopes that survival would be improved. The patient would be given very high dose chemotherapy to try to kill off the tumor cells. However, this dose not only killed the tumor but also destroyed the healthy bone marrow cells so that they could no longer function. Without functioning bone marrow cells the patient would die. Therefore, after the cancer had been destroyed, the patient would be given stem cells that had the ability to transform into functioning bone marrow cells to replace those destroyed. While at times lifesaving, this procedure was also very risky and had a pretty high complication rate. At the time, it was recommended only when there was no other choice because the cancer was so destructive that it would kill the patient without extraordinary measures. In fact, it is not done for breast cancer any more because it did not improve survival. However, at the time of this patient's diagnosis, it was performed for cancers like hers as we struggled to figure out how to beat this relentless disease.

She, however, would not even consider the chemotherapy and stem cell transplant. She told me that she did not feel it was necessary. The surgeon spoke with her, the oncologist spoke with her, and both of them said the same thing, "She is so calm about this that I wonder if she understands just how bad this cancer is."

Neither they nor I had ever seen anyone respond so serenely to this bleak diagnosis and prognosis. I was so concerned that I bluntly told her that without this treatment she would likely die—and soon. I was this direct because I wanted to make sure she really understood our fears for her.

She explained that she fully understood the diagnosis. She and her husband had both been on the Internet and had extensive information. They knew the prognosis, understood the odds, and had made the decision that she did not want the procedure.

I even brought up her young children, and I'll never forget her response. She said, "Oh, Dr. Bauman, you don't have to worry about that. I've talked this over with God, and I know that I will be alive to see my children finish school. I'm sure of this."

I was amazed. I don't think that I had ever

before encountered such absolute faith. She went on to have a mastectomy and radiation. She remained cancer free for more than three years. That was most surprising given the aggressiveness of this cancer. She has since suffered a recurrence and is undergoing treatment, but she still remains a powerful example of the intensity of the mind-body and *spirit* connection and the tremendous impact it can have on our lives.

This really was and is a most unusual case. I do not wish to imply that one should rely on faith alone for healing. She certainly did not. She did some chemotherapy, surgery, and radiation, all proven treatments. She only decided against the truly extraordinary, most risky procedure, and when the cancer recurred she began treatment once again.

I am reminded of a joke about a man who was stuck on the top of a building during a flood. He had great faith that God would save him. So when a boat came by to rescue him, he waved it off. When a helicopter hovered and offered a rope, he waved it off. He finally drowned, and when he was standing before God, he lamented, "I believed in you. Why didn't you save me?" To which God somewhat testily replied, "I sent a boat and a helicopter! What more did you expect?" So please don't think that I advocate healing by faith alone. I am constantly amazed at the wonderful advances in medicine, and I have a tremendous respect for

MARY ANN **BAUMAN, MD**

the people who design the devices and develop the treatments.

We've covered a number of different aspects of psychoneuroimmunology. We've spoken of its early days and some of the research that has been done. I've given you a few examples from my life and the lives of my patients to illustrate the practical, everyday impact of this connection.

But this is only the tip of the iceberg. I believe that researchers will continue to unlock the mystery and will eventually open this "black box" just as they did with the immune system at the end of the twentieth century. As the understanding becomes more refined, it will be easier to give patients a blueprint of how to evaluate their own mind-body connection.

Nevertheless, we're here *now* and you're tired *now,* and it's understandable that you don't want to wait. So let's continue the process of analysis, moving on to the next step.

## STEP 2: EVALUATE

Review the identification process we outlined in the first step, recalling an event from the previous 24 hours and remembering how you felt about it. Once you have incorporated this identification process into your daily routine, you can begin to evaluate your daily encounters. Remember—don't go back to old experiences. You choose a new encounter each day. That way, you are always moving forward.

*In this second step, you not only decide how the encounter made you feel but you also consider how you felt just prior to the episode. Were you happy? Angry? Rushed? Annoyed? Tired? Hungry? Scared?*

This is important because your emotional state at the time often colors your reaction to the situation at hand. That reaction will influence the choices you make. Poor choices often lead to dissatisfaction and regret, and eventually you become overextended as you try to compensate. It's a perfectly understandable reaction because the lack of satisfaction makes you uncomfortable, and the regret threatens your self-esteem so you want to "fix" it.

As I said in Chapter 1, we have a powerful need to feel good about ourselves. However, the attempt at "fixing" initiates a vicious cycle that ultimately results in exhaustion simply because you can't keep up with all the balls you need to juggle as you try to keep everyone happy. The process is tiring and drains your energy. Unfortunately, it is an all too common occurrence. Just like a baby who must crawl before walking, you must become aware of these influences before you can figure out how to put an end to the cycle. This step begins that awareness process.

Women have a great capacity to focus on fixing the immediate uncomfortable situation

MARY ANN **BAUMAN, MD**

without recognizing how much other emotions play a part in that discomfort. I am reminded of a woman in her thirties who came to see me many years ago. She told me that her husband and children were upset about her PMS. She, too, did not like the way she was reacting and felt that she needed to do something about her symptoms.

In the course of obtaining her medical history, I learned her husband was beating her. The abuse obviously disturbed her. Yet she never made the connection between this severe trauma, both physical and emotional, and the escalation of her PMS symptoms. In fact, she was quite surprised when I suggested that her marriage might be the major reason why she was irritable and upset.

Now you may wonder how she could ignore this seemingly obvious association, but I have come to realize over my years of practice that her unawareness is not unusual. Many women do overlook the role that one's emotional state plays in one's physical health. We also have a propensity to blame everything on our cycles, when, in fact, we are really experiencing a manifestation of the powerful mind-body connection.

The mind-body connection does have an impact in *your* life whether you choose to acknowledge it or not. It influences your daily encounters with loved ones, friends, and even acquaintances.

It does affect your energy because that energy is dependent on the balance in your life. If you want to maximize your energy, you must pay attention to these influences on a daily basis. So begin step two. You'll be surprised at what you discover.

# CHAPTER 3

# OH! THE CHOICES WE MAKE

If we never make the effort to analyze the choices we make, we put our energy at risk. If we never stop to evaluate the circumstances and assumptions that lead to those choices, we are likely to elicit the same unsatisfactory responses time after time. This leads us to continue to "beat our heads against the wall" in an effort to feel better about ourselves and to appease our self-esteem worries. It's a vicious cycle and it is exhausting.

We may know that a particular situation makes us uncomfortable, but we don't stop to figure out why. We just know that it doesn't feel good and we react indiscriminately. We respond to our need for every relationship to be "okay" so that we can feel "okay." A perfect example is the encounter with my colleague in Chapter 1. I kept getting negative vibes from him. So what did I do? I immediately assumed that *I* needed to change something to fix the relationship. That was a totally erroneous assumption, but it was my first impulse. What a waste of time and energy!

Likewise, if we are not aware of the thought processes that lead us to the good decisions that we make, then we lose the opportunity to nurture those healthy impulses so that we can achieve satisfying outcomes more often. Understanding our thought processes and motivations is just as important when things turn out well as when they turn out badly.

## The Myth of the Indispensable Woman

In our quest to feel good about ourselves, we often give our families more than they want or even expect. Remember the old saying, "Work will expand to fill the time allocated to it"? Substitute "needs" for "work" and you have another truism. Let me cite another anecdote from my personal repertoire.

I have always changed our bed sheets every Saturday morning as part of my weekend routine. When Lauren was about 10 years old, she went through a stage in which her room was just a mess.

I know this usually happens during the teenage years, but she was always a bit ahead of her time—for both good and bad habits! I found myself becoming irritated each time I went into her room on those Saturdays.

Finally one day I just said, "Lauren, I can't stand the way your room looks, and it makes me angry when I go in to change your sheets so I'm not going to do that anymore. You are now responsible for that job." I anticipated all kinds of hysterics, but to my surprise, she did not object. She simply took over the task.

As so often happens when I pay attention, I learned a valuable lesson. In my mind, changing the sheets was one of the tasks that *I* did for my family. It was one of the things that showed that *I* cared. It was a need that *I* met. Yet it obviously did not have that same significance for my daughter. To her it was simply a chore to be completed, and as long as I was willing to do it, she was not about to object. On the other hand, it was no big deal if I stopped.

Think about how many tasks you do each day that might fit into this category. I bet you can come up with quite a few if you are creative. Then experiment a bit. Pick one chore that's especially a hassle for you and ask someone else to do it. Don't, however, set yourself up for failure by choosing one that you know will raise objections. That's not the point of this exercise. Pick something simple.

You may be as pleasantly surprised as I was with my daughter.

Also, do not limit this evaluation process to the home only. There may be situations at work that fit into this same category. For example, in my medical office I would rewrite each patient's routine prescriptions once a year. For some of my older patients that could involve six to ten individual prescriptions that I would traditionally write out at the end of their appointment with me. Not only did this take up precious time, but my handwriting, which is never good, became less and less readable as the day went on.

Several years ago I listened to a tape on practice efficiency in which the narrator suggested that the staff write out the prescriptions before the visit and attach them to the chart. That way, all the doctor has to do is review them and sign if they are correct. I thought this was a great idea but never brought it up with my team because I assumed they were already too busy to incorporate something new. I sincerely believed that they would balk if I gave them one more task.

Imagine my surprise when, after listening to the tape, *they* suggested to me that this might be a good idea if I would be willing to try it. You would be amazed at how much time this saved for me—and as an additional bonus, their writing was legible! We've since converted to an electronic medical record, and they still print out those routine

MARY ANN **BAUMAN, MD**

prescriptions for me. Therefore, when I say to be creative, I mean it. Every task you remove from your day can add to your energy account.

Because we women are such capable nurturers, we can easily fall into the trap that we are the only ones who can adequately meet a particular need. This makes us reluctant to delegate. Instead, we take everything on ourselves and then become resentful when we are overloaded and tired. This is especially true when it comes to our children.

I remember a wonderful anecdote I heard during a talk years ago given by Marianne Neifert, M.D., who wrote an excellent book titled *Dr. Mom: A Guide to Baby and Child Care* (Neifert). She told this story about her medical partner who had just had a baby. The new mom, who was also a pediatrician, brought the infant in for a checkup. When Dr. Neifert examined her, she noticed that the baby's diaper was on backwards. She pointed this out to her partner who answered that the diaper was just fine. Dr. Neifert was puzzled and repeated her comment that the diaper was on backwards. Her partner once again replied that it was fine.

But Dr Neifert persisted, "I know that you know how to put on a diaper, and that is not on right!"

Her partner smiled, "Her dad put it on...and it is just fine." Wasn't that an emotionally healthy response? That mom was wise enough to recognize that the important issue was not the placement of the diaper, but rather that the dad was willing to take on the task. I know I have often been guilty of believing that I alone could handle a particular situation or a need involving my child. I also know there were times when I felt stressed and thought (resentfully, if I'm being honest) that the burden of responsibility for childcare fell disproportionately on me.

I have come to realize that this was largely of my own making. I set myself up to be the primary caretaker in part because I loved the role, and in part because I was meeting those frequently burdensome self-esteem needs. I was reluctant to ask for help, but that did not stop me from becoming resentful when someone did not anticipate my needs and offer to meet them. This is a common trap that ensnares many women.

## Wasting Our Energy on Unreasonable Expectations

If your personal self-esteem always depends on meeting others' needs so that they will think well of you, then it logically follows that you will become very much attuned to the needs of others. It's true—most women are quite intuitive. We anticipate, we respond, and then we expect approval and gratitude for our efforts.

However, here's what often gets us into trouble. We expect *others* to anticipate our needs

MARY ANN **BAUMAN, MD**

the same way. Now ladies, most men are simply not as good at it as we are. As we saw in Chapter 1, most learn from boyhood to define their self-esteem in ways that are not so dependent on others' approval. As a consequence, they don't generally have the same well-honed awareness antenna. They are not as intuitive. They expect us to ask if we need something, just as they do.

They don't anticipate nearly as well as we do, but that doesn't stop us from holding them to our lofty standards. The result is often an unsatisfying encounter, a no-win situation. Here's an example: You want your husband to do something for you, but you don't want to ask because that would be *selfish*—so you hint a bit. But he doesn't take the hint so you get either angry or resentful or both—not a healthy reaction!

I know it sounds simplistic, almost funny, when I put it this way. Truthfully, it would be funny if only this particular scenario was not responsible for so many relationship problems. We don't want to make our needs known, but we get angry if our mate does not anticipate them.

By the way, this reaction is in no way limited to chores around the house or family responsibilities. It is even more significant when it comes to emotional issues. He may not automatically recognize an emotional need that you have, and you might very likely interpret this as "he doesn't care." You become hurt and then erect yet another of those tiny emotional barriers that ultimately undermine the relationship.

Examples are always helpful to illustrate the point. A friend of mine was wonderfully intuitive, but she was married to a man who was not. He was a businessman and was quite successful. She became pregnant with their much-anticipated first child, but, sadly, suffered a miscarriage early in the pregnancy. She had to have a D & C, a surgical procedure to make sure that the entire placenta had been expelled, but recovered without problems and went back to work the next week. She was emotionally drained but physically fine.

Her husband had planned a reunion trip with friends for that following weekend. It had been scheduled for months, and he asked her if she wanted him to cancel. She said, "No, I'm fine." Yet she really meant, "Yes, I'm having a hard time with this, and I would like you to be here with me." Sound familiar?

You can guess what happened. He went on his trip feeling confident that she was fine because that's what she said. She stayed home feeling hurt and resentful because he didn't care enough to understand that she couldn't possibly be fine so soon after this sad event. This couple separated and eventually divorced. Now I do not wish to imply that this one episode caused their divorce. On the contrary, I am convinced that this was one of the many resentments she held onto from the many times he did not anticipate her emotional needs over the course of their relationship. She made the assumption that he didn't care many times over.

We women must make our needs known. We must understand that not everyone is as good at anticipating as we are. We must level the playing field and give others a chance to respond. Then if they really do not react appropriately, we have a right to pass judgment. If my friend had asked her husband to stay with her and he still went on the trip, then he would have been guilty as charged. Yet she never knew what he would have done had she been direct. You may argue that he was just trying to manipulate her into saying she didn't care because he really wanted to go on the trip, no matter what. That may be true, but she never gave him the opportunity so she can't be sure what he would have done.

This really is a major issue for women. Remember when we talked about ego? How often do you find yourself unwilling, even to the point of being unable, to tell someone what *you* want because you are afraid they will think you are being selfish? Instead, you hint around hoping that they will get the point. When they don't, you become angry. You know that if the situation had been reversed that you would have known what they meant without it having to be spelled out. You then interpret their lack of response as a rejection and that leads to more anger and, ultimately, resentment.

I'm pleased to say that this woman did learn from her experience and is now in a satisfying long-term marriage. She understands that her intuitiveness is not shared by everyone and realizes that she has a responsibility to avoid "setting up" her spouse. It was both a painful and valuable lesson to learn.

This was a lesson I had to learn as well. I am one of those people who anticipates others' responses with pretty good accuracy. I, too, used to be reluctant to really state my needs, but I did do a lot of "hinting." Often, I was disappointed with the result, and when I did not get the desired response, I felt unappreciated. I've worked hard on this through the years and now make it a point to state my preferences if I have them. Then I can evaluate the other person's reaction fairly. My husband jokes that I've learned this lesson *too* well, but in all seriousness, it saves me from forming resentments that can have damaging consequences. Remember, though, stating your needs or preferences does not always insure that you are going to have it your way. It simply means that you take the guesswork out of the process. Then both parties can debate the merits of the choices and find an acceptable outcome.

So what does all this have to do with your energy? Plenty. Think about how much time you waste being angry or resentful. Think about the upset to your mind-body balance. This is the key. Your level of energy is not just dependent on the number of hours you sleep each night or the number of loads of laundry you do or the number of appointments you keep. It is equally dependent on the choices that you make—choices that can either promote your balance or threaten it. You must learn to recognize your choices and challenge your assumptions if they lead to behaviors that threaten your balance.

## Recognizing Our Choices

I've often encountered women who believe that they have no choices. They believe that others are controlling the decision-making process, and they must simply follow even though it makes them unhappy. Some develop a "victim" mentality because things are always done "to them." This is devastating to one's self-esteem and energy levels, both psychological and physical.

I contend that, in reality, we usually do have choices. It's just that sometimes none of them are exactly palatable. So you say, "What difference does it make if you have no choices or just bad ones? Either way, you are forced to accept the unacceptable." But that is not true.

Understanding that there are options available makes a tremendous difference in your sense of control. Just knowing that you have choices helps you to realize that you can exert influence over your environment. Once you recognize that you have choices, you can start to explore new possibilities. Finally, making a choice takes away the sense of hopelessness that is a direct threat to your self-esteem. When you don't believe you have any control over a situation, you quit looking for ways to make it better. You subconsciously accept the limitations that others have placed on you. You *assume* that the outcome has already been determined, and you risk making a big mistake.

Here's a perfect illustration involving a young woman who just couldn't see the possibilities. She was in her late twenties and had a college degree. She was married to a man who was a few years older, and they had one child, a little girl. Her husband was extremely rigid. He controlled all of the finances, made all of the decisions, and was often emotionally abusive toward her. She suffered from many of the symptoms that frequently occur when one does not pay attention to the mind-body connection. She was depressed, had problems with sleep, and suffered from headaches and panic attacks. We discussed at length her symptoms and the emotional stress she was experiencing. She would not go to counseling because her husband did not approve and would not allow it.

After several years and many appointments with me because she did not feel well, she decided that her relationship really was not working and she did not want to be married to this man anymore. In the very next breath, however, she indicated that in spite of this conclusion, she would just have to live with this unacceptable, emotionally damaging situation. She had a child, she didn't have a job, and she had no money or skills. Bottom line, she had no choice but to stay in the marriage.

I looked at her in surprise and asked, "What do you mean you have no choice? You are a healthy, college-educated woman. There are lots of ways for you to support yourself and your child if necessary."

Initially she was quite skeptical, but over time she began to save a bit of money each week from her household account. Eventually she consulted a lawyer and finally confronted her husband. He refused to consider marriage counseling. Months later with much support from family and friends, she moved out and found a job.

I relate this story not to applaud the end of her marriage. That is always a very sad event and should never be considered lightly. My purpose is to emphasize just how blind we can become to our options. She sincerely believed she had no choice when in reality she did have a choice, but it was a scary one. She really could not imagine how she could function without the financial safety net her marriage provided. Because of this, she was willing to endure all manner of insult. Because she was convinced that she had to stay, she quit looking for creative solutions. She became, in her mind, the hopeless victim of a controlling husband. It was only when she finally allowed herself to accurately consider her options that she found a way out of that damaging situation.

Guard against this very common mistake. Try to take a 360-degree look at the problems you face, and don't be afraid to think about the tough solutions. You may be surprised at the possibilities that are open to you. Also, be aware that when you do make a choice, you have to be willing to accept the consequences of that decision. This next scenario will illustrate this point.

It involves an older patient who was unhappily married for over 40 years. She finally decided to move out and went to Georgia to live with a close cousin who had been a wonderful member of her support network for many years. She was very happy and seemed to adjust quite well to her new life. So you can understand my surprise when, after about 10 months away, she moved back and rejoined her husband who had been begging her to come home. I asked her what had prompted this decision. Had he suddenly changed? Did she now think things would be different? Had she missed him more than she expected? I was really quite curious because I knew she had not made the decision to move out hastily. She had sought counsel and had been very thoughtful and deliberate. It had not been an easy choice.

She answered my questions with the same quiet insight I had come to expect from her. "No," she said, "he has not changed." She knew things would not be different, and she really had not missed him all that much. She admitted she had really enjoyed her new life. Then why, I pressed, did she come back? She'd already done the tough stuff. She'd confronted him, told her family, and changed her household.

Her reply surprised me a little bit. She did it for financial reasons. She was concerned that this late in life she might not have the resources she would need for the rest of her life. Although she was doing fine at the moment, she wanted that security back. While I did not necessarily agree with her decision, I did respect the fact that she had made a choice that she felt was in her best interests. Then I ended the conversation with a caution, "Remember that you made this choice with your eyes open. You know what to expect from your husband. You know the limitations of this relationship, and you know that you cannot control his behavior. You can only control your own reactions."

She said she understood, but there were many times when she came back in to see me complaining about the things he did, and I had to gently remind her of her choice. She invariably smiled and acknowledged the point. She continued in counseling and, overall, was content with her decision.

These two examples illustrate both sides of the "choice" coin. Both of these women made decisions that were quite difficult and painful, but the point I want to emphasize is that they *did* have choices. Certainly, both would have preferred their marriages to be happy and fulfilling, but unfortunately that wasn't to be. Instead, each examined the options that were available and made a choice.

Figuring out your choices is not just limited to life-changing relationship issues. My wonderful friend, Cathy Keating former First Lady of Oklahoma, often tells the story of our first meeting. My nurse came to me one day and excitedly told me that someone from the First Lady's office wanted to know if Mrs. Keating could become my patient since her previous doctors were all in Tulsa and she now lived in Oklahoma City. I certainly did not hesitate. I had been impressed with the Keating family during the campaign and looked forward to meeting the First Lady whom I had only seen on television. I was also honored that she had selected me to be her doctor.

The day Cathy arrived for her appointment; I was a bit nonplussed at the well-armed State Trooper who accompanied my new patient back to the examination waiting area. I had not encountered bodyguards before, but over the years

I came to know and greatly admire these officers. They are dedicated professionals.

My nurse followed our usual routine, recording the vital signs—blood pressure, pulse, temperature, etc.—and then I entered the room to take her history. When I came to my standard question about exercise, she responded without hesitation, ticking the points off on her fingertips, "Well, I get up at 6 a.m., I work 14 hours a day, I host dinners almost every night, I always take the stairs, and I never stop moving. I'm always active."

I asked again, somewhat pointedly as she recalls, "But what do you do for *exercise?*"

Obviously, this was an exceedingly busy woman who took her responsibilities to the people of Oklahoma very seriously. I told her that if she wanted to keep such a hectic schedule and continue to enjoy the service activities she loved, then she had to find time to replenish her energy reserves. She *thought* that she was making the right decision for her situation, but realized then that she was also making the choice not to formally exercise. Cathy always laughs as she tells this story, but says that it made her stop and think—and start going to the gym!

Choices abound in your life. You make choices every day involving your relationships, your work, and even your leisure time. You must be creative and you must accurately assess your situation if you are to see the possibilities.

## Challenging Our Assumptions

When you decide to make a choice, you must carefully examine the assumptions that led you to that point so you can be certain that they are valid. You don't want to base your decisions, large or small, on faulty premises. Now that may sound obvious, but you would be surprised at how often we repeat the same mistakes because we never stop to think about whether our assumptions are correct.

Many of us know people who are divorced but who go on to marry the same type of person again (and sometimes, unfortunately, again and again). They are attracted to certain traits but do not stop to analyze whether this type of person is really what they want or need. George Santayana's observation, "Those who cannot remember the past are condemned to repeat it," could easily be changed to "Those who do not examine their mistakes are condemned to repeat them."

I faced this issue myself with the dissolution of my first marriage. I sought counseling in an effort to figure out why it had failed or, more specifically, why *I* had failed. I wanted to understand this so that it wouldn't happen again. I wanted to understand my own needs in a relationship so that I would make a better choice for myself in the future. My former husband was a good person, but ultimately not the right partner for me. So I wanted to understand what had led me to choose him. In short, I wanted to examine my assumptions about what I wanted in a life mate to see if they were valid.

It was initially very uncomfortable for me to do this because there is so much pain and guilt that accompanies divorce. However, once I got started, it turned out to be a fascinating exercise and one I still continue to this day. I still work to challenge my assumptions, to ask why I make the choices that I make. What leads me to decisions—both good and bad? Why do I do what I do? Should I continue along this path or should I change? That is the key. You *can* change things, but only if you are aware enough to know that they need changing.

A number of the examples that I have cited involve women who have made the decision to divorce, myself included. That might make you question their relevance if you are married or single. It might make you think that I am advocating that the best decision in a troubled relationship is to end it and move on. In fact, the opposite is true. The sad fact is that many potentially salvageable relationships end because both people fail to understand their motivation. They get into a vicious cycle of hurt and resentment that culminates in the decision to split because the partners see no other way to end the unhappiness.

Unfortunately, many people enter into relationships without a clear understanding of their own needs, and then they expect their partner to somehow figure out what they themselves don't know. This is a recipe for failure. The reality is that even in a fulfilling relationship there are times of stress when the outcome could go either way. Yet the partners have the commitment to find a common pathway so they make it through the risky period.

The principles we've been discussing are relevant regardless of your marital status. If you understand your motivations, your choices, and your needs, you will be a healthier partner and will have a higher chance of finding and maintaining fulfilling relationships, whether personal or business. You will be better equipped to weather the stormy periods that are inevitable.

Understand also that this examination of assumptions has to be an ongoing process because you are not a statue frozen in time. Your reactions are constantly colored by your life experiences. I'm not the same person today that I was when I married my first husband—or even when I married my second, for that matter. There is no way that you are the same person you were years ago. Life has happened. But if you make this a dynamic process, one that you do continuously, then you will be in touch with yourself. You will be routinely testing your assumptions to make sure they are still valid and you will make better choices—choices that enhance your sense of well-being, satisfy your mind-body connection, and improve your energy.

It can take a very long time before you are ready to approach your most closely held assumptions this way. They may be so deeply ingrained that you just accept them as an undeniable fact of life. I've seen this happen with young adults whose learning disabilities were not diagnosed during childhood. They simply accepted that they were not very smart or that reading was not for them. I remember one young man who was in college before his dyslexia was identified. His relief was evident when he told his mom, "I just thought I was dumb."

Another pitfall to guard against is adopting the assumptions of others. Sometimes you may accept others' assumptions into your own belief system even though you have not had the same experiences, and their assumptions are not valid for you. In spite of that, you still make decisions that affect *your* life based on *their* assumptions. You are especially vulnerable to this when it comes to the beliefs that your parents pass on to you. While it is likely that most of their viewpoints are beneficial, there is that occasional one that doesn't serve you well. The challenge (there's always a catch, isn't there?) is to sort the "wheat from the chaff," and it may be years before you are ready to do that.

Consider the case of a professional woman that I know. She was quite successful financially and yet never felt secure about her income. She always worried that it was not enough. She even knew why. Her father had grown up in a very poor household and worked hard to be successful. Because of his tough experiences as a child, he was always concerned about having enough money to meet future needs. She grew up admiring him and incorporated his concerns into her belief system. When she finally reached the point where she was willing to address her own feelings of financial insecurity, she acknowledged that the circumstances in her life were totally different from her father's. His assumptions were appropriate based on his life experience, but they were not valid for her. Yet she had accepted them for years as gospel, and they were keeping her from enjoying her success. She has now shed those adopted beliefs, but many years passed from the time she first recognized the assumptions to the time when she was willing to tackle them.

There is no statute of limitations on this process. The next step in our improvement plan will help you get started testing your own assumptions. It is the last step in the analysis phase of the plan, and it is vital to your energy restoration.

# STEP 3: CHALLENGE

In the first step of the program you got into the habit of identifying and recalling an encounter from the previous 24 hours and evaluating how you felt afterward. In the second step you began analyzing how you felt immediately before these encounters. Now that you can routinely identify your emotions at the time of an incident, you are ready to start challenging your assumptions.

*This time when you recall an incident, think for a moment about what you thought would happen in the encounter before it occurred. Then compare it with what actually did happen. In this way you are testing the validity of your assumptions. And those assumptions often determine how you will respond to a situation.*

For example, remember how my overstressed patient whose mother was about to visit just *assumed* her mother would reject staying in a hotel? That assumption made her reluctant to even suggest it as a solution to her exhaustion and stress. Or remember how I *assumed* my family did not want me to run? Because of that assumption I almost skipped an important energizing experience. We all do it.

I once had a patient who came to see me because she had spells that would periodically cause her to become weak and exhausted. Her back muscles would tighten up, and she would be very uncomfortable. I suggested counseling because she had some concerns about her aging parents and other aspects of her life. Although we were searching for physical reasons for her symptoms, I thought we could approach these other issues simultaneously.

She was reluctant at first because she thought it would be an upsetting ordeal but finally accepted my suggestion. When she came back to see me a few weeks later, she happily relayed that the counseling was wonderful, and definitely not the painful experience she had expected. Her initial assumption had been inaccurate. If she had relied on that assumption to make her decision, she would have never experienced the relief that the counseling sessions brought her.

In this chapter, we have discussed some pretty heavy-duty assumptions, such as those that come into play when you are choosing a mate. That's not what this step is about. Just like the other steps, this one is designed to make you aware of why you do what you do. It is intended to get you into the habit of analyzing your decisions and thinking creatively about your choices.

So for now, don't focus on the life-changing assumptions but rather on the small ones that influence the many decisions you make every day. You will have ample opportunity as time goes on, and you get better at the process to look at the bigger assumptions in your life. For now, keep it simple.

First you *identify* how you feel after an encounter. Then you *evaluate* how you felt prior to the episode. And finally, you *challenge* the accuracy of your assumptions. While this may sound like a lot of effort, it really takes only a few minutes of your day. In fact, it's kind of fun, especially when you begin to challenge your assumptions.

But the best part is yet to come. Now it's time to think about changing your behavior. On to the action steps!

# CHAPTER 4

# THE BARRIERS WE ERECT

How often do we make our lives more complicated and contribute to our own energy depletion? Most of us fail to recognize that this is a common occurrence. Frequently we set ourselves up for failure even when we have the best of intentions. Often we are blindly responding to a self-esteem need; in other instances we simply are not in tune with our own feelings on a particular subject. If we're serious about maximizing energy, one of the things we absolutely must do is identify and dismantle the barriers that are so firmly in place—barriers we ourselves often erect.

A barrier develops as a response to something that makes us uncomfortable. It is a way to justify our actions—and more often, our inaction! I remember reading that when someone says, "I'll try," what they really mean is, "I won't." Frequently I have found this to be true, especially when it comes to the subject of exercise. Now be reasonable, you didn't really think that I would write a book about increasing energy without discussing the "E" word, did you? Come on, I'm a doctor! Exercise—more precisely, the lack of it—is responsible for so many of our modern health problems. We're too busy, too stressed, and too tired to exercise, right?

Wrong! Exercise is one of the best energy repleters there is. What do I mean by that? I mean that exercise helps you overcome those very excuses that are keeping you from exercising.

## Replenishing Your Energy Stores

In the early 1980s, Dr. Holly Atkinson wrote a book called *Women and Fatigue* (Atkinson). In it, she suggested that each of us has a finite amount of energy. Think of it as a "bowl" of energy. There are things we do each day that take from that bowl, and there are things we can do that replenish that bowl. If we only withdraw and never refill, we will eventually come up empty. Exercise restores your energy; it helps replenish the bowl. You may be tired when you start, but when you finish you will feel energized.

I've mentioned earlier that I am a runner. I have been religiously running at least three to five times each week for over 20 years, yet there still are times when I just don't feel like doing it, when I have to force myself to get started. However, I can truthfully say that there has never been a time *after* I finished my run that I did not feel better, both mentally and physically. I always feel energized no matter what time of day it is or what's been happening in my life.

In fact, I love to run when I'm angry or stressed. I use the time to imagine confronting the person who has "done me wrong." I often compose scathing letters that will never be written, let alone sent! And when I get back, I do feel remarkably better. I'm less angry and more relaxed. That's because I have released the emotion during the physical exertion. I also run faster when I am angry so I have the added benefit of finishing my course in less time!

You don't have to be a runner to reap the rewards of exercise. In fact, it doesn't really matter what you do—walk, ride, swim, jog, dance—anything that gets your body moving for a minimum of 20 to 30 minutes at least three times every week. That's your goal. If you can only manage ten minutes at the beginning, that's a start. Go for it.

Now I know that some of the fitness guidelines recommend an hour a day, but I think that goal can be a bit daunting for someone who has not been engaged in any exercise program at all. Remember, we want to remove the barriers that set us up to fail, not erect new ones. If you can manage an hour a day, that is wonderful. But if you can't, it's better to set a less ambitious goal that you will be able to achieve. Either way, there's plenty of energy to be gained.

I chose three times a week as the minimum for a specific reason. There are a number of measurable entities when it comes to energy. One of these is a scientific term called the 24-hour energy expenditure (24EE). This is the total amount of energy you expend in a 24-hour time period, measured in kilocalories (kcal).

The 24EE is made up of three parts, which together account for all of your daily energy expenditure. These three parts are the thermic effect of exercise (TEE), the thermic effect of food (TEF), and your resting metabolic rate (RMR), which is the amount of energy you expend breathing, sleeping, sitting—simply existing. Thermic effect is a technical term that measures how much heat energy is released during a particular activity. However, 60 to 80 percent of the 24EE is accounted for by the resting metabolic rate, and you want this number to be as high as possible.

Exercise will raise your RMR, but here's the kicker: Even after you've succeeded in raising your RMR, after 72 hours without exercise, it drops back down to baseline. Yes, right back down to where you started! That's the reason you must exercise at least three times a week. In most instances, such a schedule will prevent you from allowing 72 hours to elapse between your routines. I also like a three-per-week minimum because if you don't exercise on Monday, you can still do it on Tuesday or even Wednesday and still get in your three times before the week is over.

However, I do realize that it is possible to exercise three times a week and still let 72 hours lapse between exercise days. Actually, I've done it myself. For years, I always made sure I ran three times each week, but sometimes I ended up clustering my sessions on Friday, Saturday, and Sunday, depending on my schedule. After I read the studies about energy expenditure, I altered my routine. Now I make sure that I always run on Tuesday or Wednesday as well as on the weekend. That small change resulted in an added benefit for me. By adding the midweek run, I found myself averaging four sessions a week instead of three to four. Another illustration of how small adjustments in your schedule can pay big dividends.

It's important to realize that you don't have to be an athlete to use exercise to improve your energy. I recall a patient in her late 60s who came in one day for her annual physical. I had not seen her for a year, and she said she had been feeling great. In fact, she excitedly told me that she had more energy than she knew what to do with. I was delighted and asked her what had changed. She certainly had not felt that well the year before. She said she had simply started walking, and then added that it was the best thing that had happened to her in a long time.

### "Yes, but . . ."

You probably don't doubt that exercise will make you feel better. You probably believe me when I say that it will give you energy. However, you have a million reasons why you don't have the time or inclination to commit to a program for yourself, right? I see patients every day who agree that they should exercise, but far fewer who actually do it on a regular basis.

So what can you do about your time? You are busy. There are a great many demands on you. How do you break down this barrier to your energy restoration?

I agree that it is difficult to convince yourself to exercise simply because it is good for you. I don't think that it's a very powerful impetus when you have all of the other stressors of daily life to deal with. I don't think it is easy to get into the habit of exercise. In fact, have you ever noticed how easy it is to develop a bad habit and how hard it is to develop a good one? So what's a person to do?

First of all, you need to make exercise a priority—something that you do *instead* of something else. If you wait until you have time to exercise, you will never do it. You are busy. You have more to do than hours in the day. So vow to let something else slide on the days you need to exercise. Let's face it; we all waste 30 minutes a day. And even if we don't, something could be delayed for 20 to 30 minutes without dire consequences.

This is another area where you need to be creative. Ask your husband to watch the kids for you. Take your walking shoes to the soccer game and walk around the field before, after or during, if it's really boring. Your family may balk a bit at first, but after a while they will take it in stride. In fact, I'm convinced that my family sometimes doesn't even realize that I've gone out for my run.

If having an exercise partner will get you out on those days that you decide to sleep in, then, by all means, get a partner. On the other hand, if depending on a partner means that you will skip your routine when he or she is not available, then that may not be right for you. I've often heard a patient say that she walked regularly with her husband until he stopped for some reason, and then she quit as well. Don't do that. Commit to exercise even if everyone else does not.

I feel the same way about fitness clubs. If

paying the fees will ensure that you will go regularly to get your money's worth, then by all means do it. However, if it means that you have to set aside two hours to get there, change, exercise, shower, and put your makeup on again, then you are likely not going to have the time to do it often. If that's your situation, don't choose that route. You are just setting up another barrier to your success.

Likewise, you don't have to like the exercise you've chosen, you just have to do it! I know that sounds a bit simplistic, but here's what I mean. Many will tell you that you should find the exercise that you enjoy so that you will naturally want to do it more often. While that does make sense, it does not address the countless people who, honestly, have never found an exercise they enjoy. Instead, it gives a ready-made excuse, "Oh, I'm still looking for the right thing for me."

Meanwhile, your energy is seeping away while you continue the elusive search. *Throw away your excuses*. There are dozens of tasks you do each day that you don't enjoy. You do them because they are necessary, or because they are just the right things to do. Make exercise one of these things.

I did not enjoy running for the first 8–10 years. However, I stuck with it because it worked for my lifestyle. I could run anywhere, and it didn't take a long time to complete. For years, I carried my shoes in my car so that if I found a break in

MARY ANN **BAUMAN, MD**

my schedule, I could take advantage of it. For me, a set exercise time does not work because my days begin and end at different times on different days. I sometimes have to grab an hour in the middle to get it done. You may have to be flexible like me. Or you may find that you are most successful by being inflexible—putting a definite appointment in your book or always exercising at the same time of day, such as first thing in the morning or just before bed. Take some time to think about what will work best for you, and then, as that old Nike commercial said, "Just do it."

## Excuses, Excuses

Remember my earlier lament about habits. It is not easy to develop a good habit. It will take at least six months of forcing yourself to exercise before you even have the chance that it will become a routine part of your schedule. I know that sounds like a long time, but if you recognize this at the outset, you're less likely to get discouraged. So often a patient will tell me rather indignantly that she exercised religiously for six weeks and didn't feel any better (or lose any weight) so she quit. Don't fall into that trap. Know that you will have to force yourself for those six months, and then if you are lucky, you might be "in the habit."

Another common barrier or, let's be blunt,

excuse involves the weather. You begin your walking program when the weather is ideal, but then comes the hot summer or the cold winter, depending on which part of the country you live in, and you quit. Recognize that your routine must continue whether it's raining, sleeting, snowing, or blowing. I just encountered a patient who fit this exact profile. She told me that she had been walking daily until the summer got too hot. I suggested that she do her walk in a local mall. She was surprised because she'd never thought of that simple solution.

Life's stresses can also foil your attempts at regular exercise if you are not vigilant. Often a patient will fall away from a program because of an unexpected event—someone gets sick or there is a crisis at home or work. I contend that you really need the calmness that exercise brings during these events. That's the time to do your exercise routine *more* often rather than less.

By the way, I do practice what I preach. If the world is going crazy around me, I always step up my exercise because I depend on the clarity that it provides. There are scientific studies that show that people who exercise regularly release fewer of the stress hormones during a crisis than people who don't. Wouldn't that be helpful when you are called upon to deal with the tough things in your life?

Be creative. Many times, I've run 2½ miles

in a small hotel room because I couldn't go outside. The people in the room below me may have wondered what was going on, but I completed my routine! Was it as good a workout as my usual run outdoors? No, but that doesn't matter as much as maintaining my exercise schedule. My goal, after all, is to keep that resting metabolic rate up to preserve my energy.

I remember one instance when I was in the kitchen warming up to run outside when Lauren wandered downstairs and wanted to talk. Those of you with teenagers know that you don't want to miss the opportunity to chat when they seek you out. And, if you are not available immediately, the moment is quickly lost. So I was torn. I needed to run, but didn't want to miss my chance for some mother-daughter time. My solution: I ran in the house. I traipsed through the hallways and up and down the stairs all the while talking with and listening to my daughter. Again, as in the hotel room, the workout was not quite as rigorous as usual, but who cares? I was able to accomplish both of my goals, and I felt good about it.

Once when I was counseling a patient about exercise, I was waxing enthusiastically about how you don't have to join a gym—you can just exercise at home, walk in place, do jumping jacks, etc. She stopped me with a rueful look. "Dr. Bauman," she said sheepishly, "We have a treadmill and an exercise bike at home already."

I laughed and asked her if she was using the treadmill at all and she smiled, "It makes a great clothes rack."

I have since found in an informal survey that many treadmills are being used in just this way. So much for my lecture about creative exercise. Let me just be succinct: To those of you who do have exercise equipment, use it!

## Life's Little Rewards

I have spent the last few pages trying to convince you of the importance of exercise to your energy balance. I have written eloquently (I hope!) of the benefits and the physiology of exercise and pointed out some of the barriers we so often erect. Now I'm going to talk about a reward system, and no—it's not hot fudge.

After I had Lauren, I lost the pregnancy weight, but everything did not quite go back the way it was before. If you've ever been pregnant, you know exactly what I mean! I knew I needed to exercise, but I was busy. I had a new baby, a new job, and we had just moved to a new city. It was a hectic time.

I joined the local YMCA, determined to get back into shape. This Y was a lovely facility with both a steam and sauna in the locker room. I absolutely love steam rooms, and this club even had a bunch of older magazines you were allowed to take into the steam room to read without fear of damaging them in the moist environment.

I made myself a deal. I could take a steam as often as I liked, but only after I had completed my workout. I can't tell you the number of times that what got me to the gym was not that I needed to exercise, not that I would look better, and not that I would feel better. It was that I could take a steam. It turned out to be a powerful incentive. Sometimes, my steam time was not long, maybe just a few minutes, but I always made sure that I did it. It was my reward.

Eventually I realized this reward system would work for others as it had for me so I introduced the concept to my patients: Find something that you like to do, but don't allow yourself to do it until you have done your exercise. Now to make this work, you need to choose a reward that is easily accessible and something that you enjoy regularly.

A number of my patients have been very successful with this approach. One woman confessed that she loved to surf the Internet when she got home from work. She made a deal with herself; she could not get on the Internet unless she had taken her walk. It was a good incentive for her. Another patient rigged up a reading stand on her treadmill. She allowed herself to read her novel only when she was on the machine. She was up to

45 minutes a day and more if she had a particularly good book!

You do need to be innovative to make this work. I remember a young woman who was a stay-at-home mom with two small children. She lamented, "Dr. Bauman, I am too busy. I just don't have time to exercise." I asked her if there were any television shows that she watched regularly. She said that she always watched one particular program every afternoon—it was her treat for the day. I suggested that she put her shoes on and walk in place during the first half hour of the program. That's all she had to do. She could sit and rest for the last half hour, but she could not watch the show unless she was moving for half of it. Her response? "I can do that!" We were able to find a solution that fit her harried lifestyle.

Like the self-esteem cravings we discussed earlier, these barriers to exercise can be quite sneaky. It's not that the reasons we give for failing to exercise are bogus. We truly are busy or stressed, and others really are making demands on our time. These are all legitimate issues in our lives. It's just that you must not accept the premise that these things make it impossible to exercise. You have to find a way to work around these issues instead of accepting the limitations they place on you. And don't be hard on yourself. If you find that you've been faithful to your exercise regimen for a while and then you "fall off the wagon," start again. Eventually you will be successful. I've seen it happen many times.

I also take heed from my patients' experiences. Frequently a patient will explain to me that she or he was forced to stop exercising for a short period of time, and then never got back to it. I've seen firsthand how easy it is "get out of the habit." So I personally am very careful not to fall into this trap.

You should be too. If you are lucky enough and persistent enough to get into the habit of exercise, then don't take it for granted. Keep it up. The rewards are definitely worth the effort, and you don't want to go through the hassle of having to reestablish your hard-won habit.

## Other Barriers to Tackle

So far in this chapter we have focused on exercise because it is a critical element in the restoration of your energy. You must approach your barriers to it honestly and with the intention of removing them. Remember what I said way back at the beginning of this book? Insight is not enough. You must actually change behavior if you are to be successful.

However, exercise is not the only factor when it comes to barriers that affect our energy. We often erect barriers to protect our self-esteem "sacred cows," and unless we become aware and dismantle them, we are likely to make the same unsatisfying and, in some cases, life-altering decisions again and again.

Nowhere is this more evident than in the decisions we make regarding our selection of a marriage partner. As anyone who has been through it knows all too well, an unsatisfying marriage will sap your energy quickly and efficiently. But did you know that people who are divorced are likely to select a second mate who is very much like their previous spouse? Often that's because they have never stopped to carefully analyze why the previous relationship did not work in spite of their good intentions.

For a woman, the self-esteem issues that we have been discussing can provide a powerful barrier to your selection of an appropriate mate—someone who will be able to meet your needs on a long-term basis. Think about it. If you are in your "people-pleaser" mode, your goal is to make your new companion think you are wonderful so that your immediate self-esteem needs can be met. This is especially true if you have recently been through the breakup of a relationship with all of the emotional bruising that entails. You will likely spend very little time on evaluating what you really need, relying instead on the intoxication of infatuation to convince yourself that you are really okay, and that the new man is right for you because he makes you feel better about yourself.

You may think that he is very different from your previous spouse, but unless you are willing to get beyond those initial self-esteem impulses, the likelihood that you will be attracted to the same type of person is high. You really don't want to be on your third failed marriage, wondering why there are no good men out there, before you start to approach this all too common barrier.

While I have presented this from the standpoint of marital relationships, it is by no means limited to those. You can substitute any relationship because these same principles apply. You may have a friend who abuses you in some way. It could involve your trust, your time, or even your goodwill. You end that relationship and immediately enter into another assuming it will be different simply because it is a different person. Don't assume. Take the time to understand what you want in a friendship and, sometimes even more importantly, what you don't want. Become aware of what draws you to a certain type of person and consciously decide if your criteria are appropriate. If you find that you are being seduced by unhealthy self-esteem cravings, don't give in. The effort you spend in evaluating your impulses will be rewarded with future satisfying relationships.

Another frequently hidden barrier to energy restoration involves forgiveness. Many women pride themselves on being very ready to forgive others when they do something hurtful. However, being able to successfully forgive others is fundamentally dependent on how well you can forgive yourself.

What does all this have to do with your energy? Let me give you a firsthand example. I remember one session during my divorce counseling when my therapist smiled at me and said, "You know, Mary Ann, there *is* life after divorce." That's true, of course, but when you are in the middle of the whole thing, you're really not convinced. One day I came in to my session very irate. I told my therapist I was quite upset with my mom because she hadn't told anyone that I was separated and getting a divorce. The counselor looked at me and asked pointedly, "How many people have *you* told? It's not your mother's place to tell people. It's yours."

That simple statement gave me pause. I had to admit that I was embarrassed and that I felt like a failure. After all, when I entered into that marriage, I thought it would be for life, and it hadn't worked out that way. What's more, everyone would be aware that I had failed. I realized that I wanted my mom to announce it so that I wouldn't have to. The counselor was right—it was my responsibility.

Over the course of those months, I also became aware that I was not very tolerant of my own mistakes. It finally dawned on me that if I couldn't (or wouldn't) accept that I sometimes did

MARY ANN **BAUMAN, MD**

the wrong thing, that I was sometimes selfish or hurtful, and that I didn't always make the best decisions, then I wasn't likely to tolerate the same types of behavior in others. I began to understand that when I said "It didn't matter" or "I accept your apology," I often was giving only lip service to those statements. I didn't really forgive the person; I just tucked the episode away as another hurt or resentment.

And that's what depletes your energy. It's one more barrier. Holding on to resentments—or worse, actively nurturing them—takes energy. Recall the elements of the 24-hour energy expenditure including the thermic effects of exercise (TEE) and food (TEF). Think of this as the "psychic effect of resentment." You can't measure it in calories, but it takes its toll.

When you recognize that your energy is not infinite and that you have some control over how you choose to expend it, then you won't want to waste even a small amount on old stuff. You will want to deal with the issue at the time, really forgive the person, and move on.

That's what I learned to do. I started by recognizing my responsibility in the breakup of my marriage, understanding the circumstances that led to it, and realizing that my very public failure was not the end of the world. By going through that process, painful as it was, I found myself much better able to understand how others get into circumstances they don't expect. It has made me a better spouse and mother—and even a better doctor—because now I can honestly forgive others for not being perfect. I can address the issue at hand, avoid the resentments, and move on. It was a valuable lesson.

I learned it through a divorce, but that is certainly not a prerequisite for the insight. If you find yourself holding on to resentments for long periods of time, you may want to investigate your own ability to forgive yourself. You may, like I did, demand perfection from others because you hold yourself to that impossible standard. This may be a barrier that you need to dismantle, for your energy's sake.

## Some Barriers Can Be Real Killers—Literally

We erect barriers in other aspects of our life as well, and it's not just women who do this. I have had many patients of both sexes who want to lose weight, yet repeatedly set themselves up to fail either by making the plan too complicated or expecting results too quickly. Soon they abandon their goal because it seems unachievable. I have a patient who had a bad experience when she was at a lower weight, and so every time she approaches that mark, she loses her momentum and starts to gain again. Until she acknowledges the barrier and dismantles it, she will not be successful.

Cigarette smokers are especially good at barrier building. When a patient tells me that he has to want to quit before he will work on quitting, I always disagree. You don't have to want to stop smoking; you just have to do it. As I said when we were discussing exercise, we all do many things each day that we don't necessarily want to do. But we do them anyway because it's our responsibility or simply because we should. Smoking cessation is one of those things.

If a smoker waits until the "right" time, he'll probably never quit. In stressful times quitting will be too difficult; in easier times it will simply add stress again. It's the perfect barrier—it holds up regardless of the circumstances!

Unfortunately, women are as good at this barrier as men. Women are smoking in record numbers, and it's taking its toll in lives lost to heart disease and cancer. If you smoke, this barrier is one you must tear down no matter how firmly entrenched. Your life may well depend on it. You can start by following these four steps:

- Change brands. You've obviously chosen this brand because you like it—so change it. If you get used to the new one, change it again and again and again, if necessary.

- Buy by the pack instead of the carton, and

never, ever bum a cigarette from anyone else. If you smoke a pack a day, then you must go to the store every single day. If you smoke two packs a day, then go twice. If you smoke a half of a pack daily, go to the store daily. Buy one pack and immediately throw half of the cigarettes away so that you only have enough for that day. Yes, I know how expensive cigarettes are. Yes, I know I'm telling you to waste them. Yes, I know this approach is more expensive and less convenient—that's the idea.

• Keep your cigarettes in a different location. If you keep them in your purse or pocket, put them in the glove compartment—or better yet in the trunk! You don't say you can't have one; you just make it more difficult to get it. Anyone with this habit knows that you sometimes light up without ever being aware that you did. One step on the path to quit is to force yourself to make a conscious choice each time you light up.

• Finally, pick a quit date. Studies show that people who pick a date are more successful at quitting than people who just keep cutting down. That's because you begin to psychologically prepare yourself for that date. When the day comes, throw away your cigarettes and lighters—use patches, gum, Zyban, or whatever you need.

If you miss your date, immediately pick another and try again. When I ask a patient about her quit date and she tells me that it passed and she was unsuccessful, my next question is always, "When is your next date?" Invariably she will look at me with this incredulous expression as if to say, "You mean I have to do it again?" Of course you do. The average person tries at least three times before being successful. Don't give up and don't get discouraged, no matter how many times you try. Remember, this craving did not develop in a day and won't go away quickly. But you can be successful.

One of my pet peeves is the designated smoking area in the workplace. It's almost become a social circle. You see the same people at the same time each day smoking, chatting, and relaxing. This is not conducive to giving up the habit! You need to make it uncomfortable to smoke. I tell my patients to stand in the middle of the parking lot directly in the wind or rain or heat or cold. I tell them not to speak with anyone and to smoke the cigarette and then immediately go back to work.

I know of one psychologist who tells his patients to smoke in the same place each day and not to drink a cup of coffee or do anything else that contributes to a pleasurable experience. Your goal is to make smoking a burdensome chore instead of a welcome hiatus.

As you can see, barriers crop up in many different circumstances. Some, like smoking, can even be life threatening. Others involve the decisions that we make about the most important relationships in our lives. However, many barriers are not so complicated or even that important. Still, they nip at your energy reserves and collectively add to the energy drain. It is important to get rid of them because you can't afford to waste even one smidgen of your precious energy.

The steps outlined in the previous chapters focused on analyzing your feelings and responses. Once you are in the habit of regularly identifying your emotions and will challenge the assumptions that shape your decisions, then you are ready to begin the action phase of the plan. We'll start with—you guessed it—barriers.

## STEP 4: ATTACK THE BARRIERS

Some barriers, such as the time constraints that prevent you from exercising, are obvious while others are much more cleverly hidden. In this step, you will take a two-pronged approach. You will break down those barriers to exercise while at the same time acknowledging and attacking some of the other barriers that can affect your energy.

MARY ANN **BAUMAN, MD**

It is important to work on both. Exercise is critical to the restoration of your energy. To deny that would be like ignoring the elephant in the middle of the room. So get started.

*Begin by making exercise your priority. Force yourself to get your body moving 3–4 times a week, rain or shine, stressed or relaxed, time or no time.*

As always, it's important to keep it simple. If you can't do 30 minutes, do 20 or 10 or even 5. The key is to reject any barriers in your path. Don't be critical. If you couldn't do as much as you had planned, vow to do better the next time, be happy with what you did, and move on. Set reasonable expectations. Your goal is to be successful. Don't sabotage that. If you like the idea of the reward system, concentrate on identifying that reward. Remember to choose something that is readily available, since you will be enjoying it multiple times every week.

If you will embrace exercise, you will feel a sense of power. Each time you finish your workout, feel proud—proud that you did something for yourself and that you did not let anything stand in your way at that particular time, on that particular day. It is a powerful feeling; trust me!

*However, as we've discussed, there are many other barriers that, if allowed to remain in place, will siphon off your energy. You must identify those and break them down one by one. Start with an easy one.*

If you can never get the kids out the door on

time and that makes your morning stressful, then that is an energy barrier you need to eliminate. So be resourceful and try a new approach. You might start bedtime routines earlier for yourself as well as the children, and get up a bit earlier in the morning. Maybe it would help to set their clothes out the night before, or you might find that making lunches and laying out the breakfast items before bed helps to ease the morning rush. Find a way to make it work, and if the first attempts fail, don't give up. Try again.

Be careful to choose barriers that you do, in fact, control. When you select something that is beyond your scope of influence, you are setting yourself up for failure. That is not what this step is about. For example, if you apply for a new job that requires a master's degree and you have only a bachelor's, it doesn't matter how well you prepare and present yourself. You are not going to get that job. On the other hand, if you decide that not having that master's degree is actually the barrier, and you choose to remove it by enrolling in a master's program, then you are taking a proactive approach and addressing that which is under your control. Even though that decision may not represent a quick solution, it might be the appropriate one for you.

As I said, all barriers are not monumental so begin by actively looking for the small ones that cause annoyances, irritation, and delays in your day. They are there; you just have to begin to recognize them. Many can be eliminated, but only after they have been identified. Each may be small, but together they will take a cumulative toll on your energy reserves. Once you start this process, it will become easier and easier to see the barriers. Ultimately, you want to get to the point where you can avoid setting them up in the first place.

It's always advisable, however, to have a few successes under your belt before you tackle some of the most difficult ones, usually those that involve the important people in your life. Don't rush it. Remember, this step is part of a long-range plan that all fits together. It is designed to help you to gradually change the way you approach your life situations so that you can avoid the traps that sap your energy.

You must still continue the analysis steps on a daily basis because each step builds on the foundation set by the others. It is through identifying and evaluating your reactions and then challenging the assumptions that led to those reactions that you will find the barriers to attack. Then, as happens with exercise, you'll do more than simply stop the loss of energy. You will actually be able to increase the amount of energy at your disposal.

# CHAPTER 5

# BE GOOD TO YOURSELF

I n the last chapter, we talked briefly about using little rewards to reinforce the exercise habit. In this chapter, we'll look at the subject of rewards in more detail. By now it's probably obvious to you that I am a big believer in reward systems. They are the icing on the cake, a little ray of sunshine in a harried week. They can be very effective when we want to stimulate a change in behavior as in the exercise example. Just as important, a reward can be a wonderful source of energy in its own right. A reward is an energy repleter, and we certainly need as many of those as we can find!

In spite of this, however, many women

never truly reward themselves. Many of us don't even take the time to figure out just what kind of rewards would give us pleasure. We are so busy taking care of others (too often because we are blindly responding to self-esteem needs) that we never stop to figure out what would make us happy.

So part of finding your energy is finding your rewards. Yes, that's what I said—*finding* them, as in *looking for* them. This is an active process, and trust me, it's not always as simple as it seems. Of course, it's easy to figure out that a trip to Tahiti would make you happy, but that's not what I mean. A big vacation may be a great escape for a short time, but it's a one-time event. I'm talking about the long haul. I am challenging you to look for the small things, the everyday things that are easily accessible and give you pleasure.

## Simple Pleasures

As always, my patients provide great illustrations. One woman told me that once a week she locks herself in the bathroom, sets candles around the tub, and takes a long, luxurious soak in a bath filled with scented salts. Doesn't that sound inviting? She reads or just relaxes, and her husband and children know that this is her time—no interruptions, no phones, just time alone. She told me that this recharges her batteries. I was impressed. It's simple, accessible, and inexpensive, even for the most budget conscious. What's more, here was a woman who was in touch with her mind-body connection. She found a way to meet her own needs, to reward herself without seriously infringing on the time needs of her family. I thought it was a great idea.

Another example of a simple pleasure: About once a month, a friend and I meet for lunch on a Friday afternoon. We go to a wonderful local sushi place, have a delightful meal, and just decompress. We started out meeting once every couple of months, but shortened the interval because it was so therapeutic for both of us. We talk about everything—and nothing. Mainly, we just relax together. I think this represents a simple way to protect our energy.

Do you have a friend with whom you'd love to spend a little extra time? It doesn't have to be someone you know well. It might be a person you'd like to know better. In fact, my friend first approached me about lunching together. We had known each other professionally and she called me one day to ask if I'd like to join her. Our personal friendship grew from this pleasant social encounter.

I'm so glad she took the initiative because it's not likely I would have made that first call. We had worked together on a few projects, and I always thought she was neat, but I probably would have missed this opportunity. Sometimes, someone else provides you with your reward. Just be sure you don't ignore it!

By the way, if you do decide to try this with one of your friends, you can expect to feel just a bit guilty at first. I know I did. After all, I did have work that I could have been doing. For a doctor, there is always paperwork waiting, but this is one of those times when you should do what I did and ignore those feelings. Realistically speaking, whatever you would have done during this time can likely wait. If it can't, you've obviously chosen the wrong day; so reschedule. Now, if you find yourself always canceling, you need to reexamine your commitment to this endeavor.

In my case, I know the paperwork will be there tomorrow. I take care of anything with any urgency to it and then I go. It works best for me to schedule these interludes well in advance because I know that if it is on my calendar, it is much more likely to become a reality. However, you may find that a more spontaneous approach works better for you and your friends. Experiment a bit, and, remember, it doesn't have to be anything fancy. You can decompress at each other's homes, the local McDonald's, or a nearby park. The key is to just take the time. You'll find yourself eagerly anticipating each visit—I still do, even though we've been doing this for years.

## Make It a Healthy Habit

Taking a little extra time for oneself is not something that most women do well. This is often quite obvious at work. All of us have deadlines to meet, that big project to complete or presentation to give, and we push to complete the task. Yet when it is over, what do we do? Do we take a break, slow down for a day, maybe take one of those long lunches, or come in a bit later in the morning? No, we scramble to catch up with what we didn't do during the crunch time. Am I right?

I once gave a talk at a seminar in Milwaukee and met a woman who faced exactly this situation. She had been extremely busy making all of the arrangements for the event, and then was leaving the next day to accompany her husband on an out-of-state trip to see his doctors for a serious medical condition. However, she had arranged to take a day off when she returned. What a smart thing to do! She told me how much she was looking forward to that time. She intended to meet her son for lunch and reveled in the fact that she would have the day to herself. I thought it was another wonderful example of a simple reward.

Try to find a way to schedule downtime into your own life. Most people eagerly plan their big vacations, but never stop to realize how therapeutic it can be to take an occasional day off—for no specific reason. If your job or workplace does not allow you the flexibility to build some free time into your schedule, then think seriously about taking a vacation day, or even part of a day, to refresh yourself. You'll be surprised how eagerly you look forward to that time. It will provide a respite from your busy schedule.

If you have a job where time off is limited or restricted, don't give up. You can still find your relaxation during your nonworking hours. I know, I know. You have so much to do that that is not an option. Not true. It doesn't have to be a huge time commitment. Just give yourself a break, even if it's only for an hour once or twice a week. Trust me, you will be more efficient and feel less burdened if you will try this approach.

I always admire people who take a day off for their birthdays. It's another nice way to pamper oneself and acknowledge a special day, although once a year is not enough. You must schedule some downtime regularly if you want to be successful at replenishing your energy reserves.

Finding this time for yourself is especially challenging if you don't work outside of the home. Those in the workforce might assume that you have total control over your schedule, but you know that is simply not true. Your job has no defined start and stop times. Even bedtime is a question if you have little ones! That means that you are essentially on call 24 hours a day, seven days a week. Talk about an exhausting schedule.

It is imperative that you take some time off; otherwise, the sacrifices you have made and the joy that you felt when you made the decision to stay home will turn into resentment, which ultimately results in wasted energy. Believe me, in your challenging situation, you cannot afford to waste that precious commodity.

You will have to be especially creative. Since your job responsibilities and hours are not well defined, there is the distinct possibility that you will never have an obvious break. You will have to build relaxation time into your schedule. I have recommended "Mother's Day Out" to many stay-at-home moms. If that's not financially feasible, then consider an arrangement with another mom so that you watch each other's kids periodically to give each of you a chance to recharge your batteries.

You'll notice that I am quite specific when I address women who are not in the workplace as "women who do not work outside of the home." Clearly, women who choose to stay at home do have jobs and work hard. The distinction is that no one is paying them a salary for their efforts. In fact, frequently the family sacrifices some of the amenities that that second income would bring because both the husband and wife are committed to this concept. If you've made this choice, don't assume that the satisfaction will be enough. Make a break happen and do it regularly.

I compare this whole process to what happens when a patient loses blood and becomes anemic. We give them iron to build the blood count back up. It will usually take six weeks for the blood tests to get back to normal. This means that they are no longer anemic and will feel better. However, we must continue the iron replacement pills for at least six months after that to replace the iron stores in the bone marrow. If we don't, then they can easily become anemic again because as red blood cells wear out, there will not be enough iron available to make new ones. In other words, the patient will have no reserves.

This is exactly what happens if you don't pay proper attention to your own energy. Even as you take care of the immediate problem, you must focus on your long-range reserves so that you are ready for the energy demands that are inevitable in your busy life.

It is also very easy to let your family needs take up all of your after-work hours and your vacation time as well. You end up taking time off to take the kids to the doctor or dentist or... whatever. You name it and you are doing it. While many times this is necessary and unavoidable, try to find another way to accomplish the task from time to time. Maybe your husband could take off occasionally and stay with the kids when they are sick or schlep them off to the appointment.

Remember, you'll never know if he's willing if you don't ask.

I know of one corporation that instituted a new policy that penalized employees if they exceeded a certain number of unexcused absences during the year. I overheard one of the employees remarking to another, "Well, my husband will just have to stay with Sarah sometimes when she is sick." Don't wait for such an ultimatum. I know that you love doing for your family, but don't make the mistake of sacrificing yourself and your energy because eventually it will wear you down. The best thing you can do for your family is to take care of yourself.

This is even more pertinent if you do choose to stay home. One of the likely reasons for that decision was to be there to take care of the children and the household. Consequently, you may feel guilty if you take time for yourself because then you are not "doing your job." Remember, no one in the workplace works day and night without a break. If they try, then everyone expects burnout, and while many women don't want to acknowledge it, burnout also occurs at home. If you let that happen, the consequences to your energy and to the well-being of your family are significant.

I am always reminded of the instructions given when you are getting ready to take off on a commercial airliner. The flight attendant instructs that in the event of a loss of cabin pressure you are to put the oxygen mask on yourself first and then those for whom you are responsible. That's because they know that if you are without oxygen, you will not be able to take care of others. The same thing applies in your personal life. If you are without energy, you will not be able to meet the needs of those who depend on you. Think about it—and take a break!

## Being Good to Yourself

Another type of reward involves pampering yourself: facials, massages, manicures, pedicures, etc. The lists of available services are extensive these days. Local spas are everywhere, and depending on your budget, these may be regular events or periodic pleasures. I get a facial every 4–6 weeks and have been doing this for more than ten years. I think it has made a difference in my skin, but that's all subjective. What really matters is that I have given myself permission to spend time and money on myself.

This is where we often hit an impasse. We are very willing to splurge on our kids or our spouses, but not on ourselves. Of course, you have to be realistic about budget constraints, but don't be afraid to add taking care of yourself into the equation.

At our office, we gave out small rewards periodically throughout the year for a job well done. We had interoffice contests and the winner was given movie tickets, bath salts, or sometimes a certificate for a manicure or pedicure. One of our employees, a single mother, said she especially enjoyed the manicures and pedicures because she had to use them on herself. If she had just received a mall certificate, she would likely have spent it on something for her kids. I thought she made a very good point. You might consider this in your own situation. Inexpensive rewards can pay great dividends for both the recipient and the giver. We all need to be appreciated.

## When Doing Good Becomes a Burden

Ignoring one's own needs will result in a loss of energy both directly and indirectly. We've been focusing on some of the direct consequences, but there are indirect ones as well. Think about this all too common scenario: You respond to everyone's demands on your time. You do this because you love your family, you love your friends, and you love to volunteer. You do this because doing for others makes you feel good about yourself and your self-esteem soars when others appreciate you. You continue to do this even though you know that you are overloaded.

However, after a while—and this may be years for some women—you begin to feel less appreciated. You feel less joyful. Others don't seem to recognize your efforts as openly as they used to. So what happens? Resentment sets in. Suddenly, you find yourself comparing how much you do versus someone else. Your irritation begins to show. You fly off the handle when your kids ask you for something or you're asked to chair a committee or your boss tells you about the next deadline. You feel used and overwhelmed, and you start to get angry at even the slightest hint of disapproval. Now your organization is no fun; you don't even like the people with whom you volunteer. To add insult to injury—your loved ones are really getting on your nerves!

When you reach this point, even the enjoyable things in your life become a chore. They simply represent more demands on your time. This, unfortunately, is the all-too-common result of not being good to yourself, of not factoring your own needs into your daily roster. You'd be surprised how often you can defuse this situation before it ever reaches the end stage by just being aware of those needs and of what will give you pleasure in your life.

Sometimes when I'm giving a seminar, I ask the participants to engage in a little exercise. I ask them to write down five energy depleters in their life. Everyone grabs their pencils and writes furiously. They are finished in no time. I then ask them to list five energy repleters. Most women pause, look around, chew on the eraser, and generally look perplexed. It takes quite a bit longer to complete this portion of the exercise. Then I throw in the kicker—take out every energy repleter that has to do with taking care of someone else. You can guess what happens; most women's lists shrink down to next to nothing. Let me reiterate what I said at the beginning of this chapter; we are not good at identifying our own needs, let alone our own wants.

We mistakenly think that keeping everyone else happy and satisfied will keep us happy and satisfied. And while I really don't want to discount the satisfaction of taking good care of one's family, I want you to realize two important points. First, you have to do it for the right reasons, and second, it can't be the only thing in life that gives you pleasure. For me, being a good wife and mother is the most important thing I do and is by far the most rewarding part of my life. However, I am careful to understand that I must have other outlets because being consumed by the needs of my family is not healthy for me. If I want to retain the joy, I have a responsibility to make certain that the things I do for my family do not become a burden.

Only I can control that. I know that sounds pretty definite, but for some aspects of everyone's life, it is true. For example, if the reason you volunteer to make three dozen cookies for your daughter's school is because you love to bake and baking is a creative outlet for you, then that is wonderful. On the other hand, if you really don't have the time or inclination to bake, but you do it anyway because that's what the other mothers do and you don't want to be "shown up," then that's a wrong reason. You are responding once again to those self-esteem "everyone has to think I'm wonderful or I'm not" routines that can be so devastating to your energy pool.

So what if everyone else bakes? The kids will likely enjoy the store-bought cookies just as much, and even if they don't, so what? It really will not affect their future development, and if it gives you a little extra time to take care of yourself, then your whole family will benefit. Remember that old, rather sexist saying, "If mama's not happy, ain't nobody happy."

The concept that good things can become burdensome reminds me of an encounter I had with one of my patients. This woman is very active. She is well beyond retirement age, yet still continues to work full time and loves it. She had tried to go part-time a couple of years earlier but was bored. She also does volunteer work for several organizations and, to top it all off, has had major surgery within the last couple of years. During our conversation, she admitted that she thought she was too busy and it was taking a toll. She was feeling somewhat anxious and was not sleeping well at night.

We talked about her options, either to cut back on work or on the volunteer activities. I asked her if financially she could afford to decrease her working hours, and she said that that would be no problem. I then asked her about giving up her volunteer "jobs." She responded plaintively, "But I love to do that!"

Something had to give. She had rightly analyzed her situation, yet was reluctant to take the next step and initiate a plan to relieve the anxiety. Both work and the volunteer activities were positives in her life. Both gave her satisfaction, but that still did not change the reality of the situation. Unless she altered her schedule in some way, her anxiety and sleeplessness and all of the discomforts that go along with those two conditions would likely get worse. She ultimately decided to speak with her boss about cutting back on her hours so that the combination of her job and volunteer activities would more closely approximate a regular 40-hour workweek. Sometimes, compromises are necessary and therapeutic.

## Getting Professional Help

I have referred to counseling and counselors a number of times throughout these chapters. If you suspect that I am a believer in the benefits of counseling, you would be correct. As I mentioned earlier, I've participated myself and found it to be intellectually stimulating and emotionally rewarding.

But I have also realized through the years that while often, through sheer force of will, I can get someone to make an appointment and go to see the counselor, I cannot make them benefit from the experience unless they are ready and open to it.

That may sound obvious, but believe me, it was not all that clear to me for a long time. As doctors, we are used to telling people what they need. We give advice and expect patients to heed that advice so that they will feel better. So when it would become apparent to me that a patient had some issues that could easily be resolved with a little expert help, I would make that suggestion—sometimes forcefully. I would say to myself, "If I can only get her (or him) to go, surely she/he will become engaged in the process and like it."

I've been wrong about that many times. I still try because I'm not one to give up easily since I do so strongly believe in the impact that the mind-body connection has on our day-to-day lives. When I encounter someone whose physical symptoms literally scream emotional upset, I always approach the subject of counseling and its benefits. Nowadays, however, if the person is completely closed to the idea, I don't push it quite as hard as I did before. I've realized that it does take a certain amount of ego strength—some confidence in yourself—to be willing to scrutinize your behaviors with someone else.

I remember a patient many years ago who

had a successful family business, but who found her life was not satisfying because of the very issues we have been discussing throughout this book. She could not keep everyone happy, and she was running herself ragged trying to do just that. She was exhausted and came to see me often looking for a physical reason for her symptoms. We did all of the requisite tests and found everything normal on numerous occasions over the course of several years' time. After I became convinced that there was no direct illness causing her fatigue, I spoke with her about her emotional state. I suggested that a counselor could help her to set some boundaries in her relationships with family and friends. I discussed the evidence implicating the mind-body connection with overall good health. I told her that seeing a counselor did not mean that I thought she was "crazy." Yet she would have none of it. In fact, I have always remembered her response.

"Dr. Bauman, it is a question of ego."

I looked at her puzzled, "You mean that you don't have much?"

To which she replied, "Oh, no. I have too much to consider seeing a counselor."

That statement was amazing to me because, in my experience, it is the people with the healthiest egos who are able to recognize when they could use some help in sorting out a problem. For this woman, however, counseling represented a failure and branded her as not being able to handle her own issues. There was also an underlying fear that counseling would somehow make her different, that it would change her personality. Although I reassured her that this would not happen and that any changes she made would be by her own choice, she just could not see it.

Her sentiments are not all that unusual. In fact, I have heard such fears repeated often. I think some of it comes from a bygone age when psychiatry was focused on disease processes such as schizophrenia, severe depression, and other behaviors that indicated underlying complicated diseases. Although this lady was not elderly, such feelings are especially common among older people. Many over the age of 65 remember the era of shock therapy (which is still used on occasion today but only for limited, severe indications.) They remember when a depressed family member just "went away" for a period of time and then came back with very little explanation of what happened during the absence. They remember that "crazy" relative or neighbor who had to be institutionalized. Psychiatry was "messing with the mind," and there was a true stigma attached to those who needed help in this area.

Times have changed. Just as with other fields of medicine, the whole science of mental health has advanced. Medications are now available that often enable even the most seriously afflicted to live a reasonably normal life in mainstream society—something that was improbable even in the 1970s. Psychiatrists today frequently use their expertise for medication adjustment, working in tandem with a counselor who does the therapy.

However, when I recommend counseling, I'm not talking about life altering illnesses. I suggest counseling, as in this woman's case, when the established patterns of behavior start to cause more pain than comfort, when "business as usual" leads to unhappiness or physical symptoms. A talented counselor acting as a trained observer can offer alternative solutions that the patient, no matter how intelligent, has not considered. It is a strength, not a weakness, to recognize that someone else might have expertise from which you might benefit. It is always interesting to me that patients are perfectly willing to take pills to relieve symptoms, but if I suggest tackling the underlying issues, they immediately shy away because they "should be able to do it themselves."

I do recognize that when a patient is in a crisis, he or she is more likely to seek help because the pain is so great. Therefore, I always recommend counseling during these times. I know that it will help with the immediate pain, but I always hope that the patient will become intrigued with the process of self-discovery and will actually continue beyond resolution of the initial trauma. During the most painful interludes in our lives—death of a family member, divorce, loss of job, or some other monumental event—our usual defenses are down. The usual coping methods prove inadequate. Often it is during such times that we are most willing to look critically at the circumstances that brought us to this point and then change our behavior.

These kinds of circumstances can jumpstart the process. That's certainly what happened for me. My divorce was a watershed event in my life. I started counseling because I was in such pain. I was embarrassed to admit that my marriage did not work. I was worried about my decision, and I was scared. I have since come to realize that these are very usual reactions, but at the time, I felt I was the only one who had ever experienced quite this depth of emotion. It's somewhat like having a baby. Even though millions of women have done the same thing, at that moment, you feel you are the only woman who has had this powerful experience.

My initial foray into the world of counseling, however, taught me another valuable lesson: You must find the right counselor; otherwise, the experience will not be beneficial for you. I started with one person who came highly recommended by someone I trusted, but he was the wrong therapist for me. Instead of coming away with hope and determination, I left each session feeling more and more discouraged. Thank goodness others pointed this out to me, and I made a change. I knew immediately that the second person was right for me.

MARY ANN **BAUMAN, MD**

She made me challenge my assumptions, she gave me homework, but most important, she gave me hope.

I also credit her with starting me on my journey of self-discovery. After I got through the initial trauma, I continued counseling because I was learning so much about my motivation, my decision-making processes, and my behavior. I tried out new approaches and found out what worked and what didn't. I began to evaluate my relationships with family and friends to determine what was healthy and what was not. Slowly, I realized that I was a pretty solid person, but like everyone else, I had some blind spots. There were times when I acted automatically just because I had always done it that way without much thought as to whether the outcome made me happy.

This is when I really started to change some things that I did not like about myself, but which I had been either unaware of or afraid to tackle. I began the process of analyzing my actions and looking at my decisions through a whole new filter. Was I acting out of healthy motivation, or was I responding to a fear or hurt or slight, actual or perceived? It was a wonderfully liberating experience, and it is a process that I continue on a daily basis.

I don't wish to imply that it was always easy, however. Sometimes I found things that I was not proud of—behaviors that were petty, irritating, or stimulated by less than admirable motivation. These I had to change because ultimately, not only did they affect my sense of well-being, they also took energy, energy that was far too precious to waste. Unfortunately, it was not a one-time deal. I still have to put my behaviors through a "healthy" filter to be sure that I don't slip back into energy-draining patterns. It's a dynamic process. Counseling was beneficial for me. The circumstances were right and the timing was perfect. The process of analysis that I began so many years ago has made me a better wife, mother, and doctor. Yet it took a new approach, and that is a perfect segue to the next step.

## STEP 5: EXPLORE AND EXPERIMENT

In earlier steps we learned to reflect on a significant encounter, good or bad, every day. In this step we go a bit further—in two phases, actually.

*First, ask yourself, what if you could go back and relive one encounter from your day? If the incident was negative, is there anything you could have done differently to elicit a more positive outcome? If it was positive, can you pinpoint why? What action or reaction on your part elicited the response?*

For example, if today's encounter was a disagreement with a loved one, it's likely that a chance remark triggered a whole cascade of

MARY ANN **BAUMAN, MD**

mounting emotions, eventually culminating in a full-blown argument. What if you had handled the initial remark differently? What if you had recognized the pattern earlier and short-circuited the back-and-forth escalation? While you cannot control another person's behavior, a fact that many of us are loathe to accept, you can control your own reactions and that has a direct influence on the outcome.

Think of how often a negative encounter happened because you were stressed from work, angry with someone else, or maybe just plain tired. Is it possible that if you had handled the initial actions differently, the outcome might have been more satisfactory?

Be good to yourself, though. You must also recognize those times when you handled a situation well and were rewarded with a pleasant response. Visualize how easily such an encounter could have turned sour if you hadn't demonstrated the wisdom and foresight to handle it smoothly. Your goal is to take those behaviors that are healthy and nurture them, while those behaviors that resulted in unhappiness can be changed.

*Now for the second phase. It's time to try out new approaches. Armed with your ongoing assessment, and having thought of a number of new ways to handle situations, you are ready to start experimenting. But now, rather than reviewing an episode that has already occurred, you choose an upcoming interaction. Try to set the scene, analyze the factors that will influence you, and visualize possible outcomes. Then use the healthy behaviors that you've previously identified to encourage a positive result.*

Let me give you an example. You've realized by now that I adore Lauren, but like mothers and daughters everywhere, we often clash. One of my joys when she was in middle school was to drive her to school each morning, but unfortunately, we often argued the whole time.

This made me very uncomfortable, and I decided that something had to change. I went through the assessment steps and realized that when I felt rushed in the morning, I had much less tolerance for my daughter's preteen ways. I would let my exasperation show, which led to anger on her part, and we were off and running headlong into another conflict. Lauren promptly forgot the whole episode as soon as she entered the school, but I was bothered all day.

So here's what I did: Recognizing that time pressure seemed to be the inciting factor, I got up ten minutes earlier, spoke with Lauren about leaving slightly earlier, and set the stage for a more leisurely morning drive. Even when we didn't quite meet our scheduled departure time, we were still earlier than before, and there was no longer a need to rush. Lauren still exhibited those frustrating teenage quirks, but now I found myself better able to cope and respond without becoming irritated. We still clashed at times, but those occasions became the exceptions not the rule.

Not every plan will work as well as this one did, of course. Still, if I had not taken the time to assess my own feelings, identify the problem, and change my behavior, I would have had very little opportunity to change the outcome.

If your first plan doesn't work, pick another encounter with the same person and go back to the drawing board. Or take on an upcoming meeting with another individual and try again. You will learn that through trial and error, you can be successful just like those little boys we talked about in the first chapter, who learned while doing puzzles with their fathers. You build self-esteem one encounter at a time.

Two important cautions accompany this step: First, be honest with yourself as you do the exploration and experimentation. After all, you are the only person in the audience. You are not trying to impress anyone else.

Second, and even more important, don't overestimate your own role. It may sound as if I am suggesting you can always control the outcome of a situation if you handle it properly. Nothing could be further from the truth. Remember my encounter with my boorish colleague? No matter what I did, I could not gain his approval. So I had to change my behavior and move on. I had to recognize that his approval, or the lack thereof, had no effect on my performance.

One of the most valuable skills we can learn is to willingly take responsibility for our own behavior, but not the behavior of others— good or bad. The challenge is to recognize what is yours to take. It becomes easier when you learn to focus objectively on your performance. That will happen when your self-esteem is no longer at risk whenever someone even hints at disapproval or when you *think* they are hinting at it.

Once again, you must keep up this process until it becomes second nature to you. That is, you must continue to evaluate your encounters to see if they could have or should have been handled differently, and you must acknowledge those that go well. This is a critical step on your road to energy restoration.

In this step, be sure to explore and experiment with rewards as well. Take the time to figure out what gives you pleasure. Find those rewards that "make your day" and then indulge on a regular basis. You must do something for yourself at least once a week. Therefore, make certain that some of your rewards are realistic and conducive to that.

# CHAPTER 6

# LIMITS CAN BE LIBERATING

We have focused a great deal of attention in the preceding pages on looking at our motivations, our relationships, and ourselves in a different way. I've tried to make the mind-body connection personal and relevant to you. Above all, I've encouraged you to develop a different filter for analyzing the events that have shaped your life so that you can better understand the significant toll that your quest for self-esteem comfort can take on your energy. If you are systematically following the steps, then you are beginning to answer the question, "Why do I do what I do?" At this point, you should not be discouraged, but rather, you should be feeling more comfortable with the analysis and experimentation process.

So now let's turn our attention to boundaries. I like boundaries. They allow me to know where I stand and to let others know that as well. I used to think that boundaries kept me from reaching my goals. I now know that they help me to realistically set my goals so that I can be successful. In addition, there is no better boost for one's self-esteem than feeling that sense of accomplishment for a job well done.

## Whose Boundaries—Yours or Theirs?

It is important for you to understand that when I speak of boundaries I am not referring to limits that are designed to discriminate against someone. These may involve gender, race, religion, or any of a host of other illegitimate reasons inappropriately used to judge one's capabilities. I grew up in the early days of feminism and have experienced gender bias firsthand. I still see it today, although thankfully to a lesser extent. Being the mother of a bright young woman, I do worry about the situations she will face. Yet I know that having to prove my worth over and over again, having to prove that I was not a "flash-in-the-pan," did give me a sense of purpose that was valuable.

When I entered medical school in the 1970s, there was the expectation that as a woman your performance would be scrutinized. There were many who still felt that most women would not be able to keep up with the rigors of a doctor's life and would be unwilling to make the necessary, long-term commitment. As a result, I understood that my success or failure could directly impact the women who followed me. We women needed to be better prepared, more gung-ho, less tired, and more enthusiastic than our male colleagues so that everyone would realize that allowing more women into medical school was the right course.

I think this attitude was beneficial for me because it gave me a higher sense of purpose. I was not just pursuing my own goals; I was also improving the situation for those who followed. That was almost 30 years ago, and today women have achieved parity in medical school admissions. Young women doctors no longer have that same need to prove themselves for the sake of others who follow. It has become a nonissue. While a part of me acknowledges that this is what we were working for, another part feels that these young doctors are missing out on a valuable experience.

Certainly, gender challenges remain. For example, as my daughter was reading this passage over my shoulder, she said she felt the same way about the issues that will face our first woman president who will likely be judged not only as a leader, but also as a woman. Glass ceilings still remain, and no woman should compromise her goals because someone else tells her she can't do it.

At my hospital, we do a program for high school students called "On Your Own." We discuss with these young people the health challenges they will face as they leave their parents' homes and strike out into the world as adults. For years we had a wonderful motivational speaker who became pregnant when she was only 15, yet eventually earned a Ph.D. in engineering. She related her experiences and chronicled the number of people who told her she couldn't or wouldn't succeed. She encouraged the young women to set high goals, to believe in themselves, and to do the hard work necessary to make their dreams come true. It was and is a powerful message and always resonated well with the students.

So when I say I like boundaries, you must understand the context of my statement. The boundaries I'm referring to are the ones we set ourselves. As we have seen, if we run ourselves ragged to meet the expectations of others simply to feed our hungry self-esteem demons, then we will not feel satisfied. We will feel that others are taking advantage of our good will, and that leads to resentment, overextension, and ultimately, energy loss. This is where limits can be liberating. By setting reasonable limits or boundaries on what we demand of ourselves and what we allow others to demand from us, we free ourselves from the

MARY ANN **BAUMAN, MD**

energy-depleting effects of unreasonable expectations.

## The Foundation for Good Boundaries

Good boundaries come from an understanding of our own motivations and needs. They come from knowing what we require to make us happy. Therefore, in order to set the type of boundaries I am suggesting, you must do some soul-searching because most of us do not automatically know what it will really take to make us happy.

For example, we often think we might find happiness in different relationships, better jobs, or new cities, but these are often not the answer. Even if we achieve them, they may not do the trick. That's because we don't understand our feelings, reactions, and motivations. We've not become proficient in the analysis steps outlined in the previous chapters so we erroneously think that a location change will magically lead to happiness. This is called a geographic escape, and I see it happen frequently with patients, colleagues, employees, and friends. I also confess that, when stressed, I still fight the urge myself!

The reason a geographic escape doesn't work is that you still have to take *you* with you, and that's the problem. Let me give you an example involving a woman who has been my patient for years. She had not been happy with her life for some time. One day she came in and said she had made a decision: She was moving across the country and was going to enroll in a vocational school to learn a new skill. When I asked her why, she said she needed a change, and she thought this would make her happy.

It was clear to me that this was an impulsive decision made because she was feeling unsatisfied. She did not have a well-thought-out plan. We discussed this on several different occasions and eventually she reconsidered. Ultimately, she decided not to sell her home, give up her support systems, and move. She did, however, get into counseling and worked hard to determine her true happiness needs.

Another patient of mine found himself unsatisfied with his life in his mid-40s. He was being heavily recruited for a position similar to his present one, but located in another state. After much soul-searching, he decided to make the move. He put his house on the market, enrolled his son in a new school, and off the family went. His wife and son adjusted well to the new town, but he did not. Less than a year later, he moved them back causing a great deal of turmoil for all involved. What's more, his previous job was no longer available. This was a classic case of a geographic escape, and it illustrates so well why it doesn't work. Rather than tackle the reasons for his unhappiness, he decided that a new environment would solve all of the problems. Of course, he was wrong. Sadly, as of today, he still has not approached the real reasons for his dissatisfaction. Until he does, I predict the turmoil will continue for his entire family.

Contrast the above situations with another involving one of our former employees. This young woman had worked for many years for a local company. Then during an economic downturn, she was laid off. She was given a severance package and used those resources to go back to school to become a nurse. She loves her new profession and is wonderfully enthusiastic and skilled. She took what was a tough and unexpected setback and turned it into an opportunity, but she would not have been so successful if she had not taken the time to understand what would truly make her happy and satisfied. She illustrates perfectly that old saying, "When life gives you lemons, make lemonade!"

Another patient was faced with a difficult situation involving chronic pain after an accident. She had sustained shoulder injuries and was unable to go back to her old job. She was quite discouraged about this, which was ironic since she had always complained that she hated her work and wanted to do something different. One day I asked her why she wanted things to be back the way they were even though she had not been all that satisfied with her previous life situation. She paused, became thoughtful, and then laughed saying, "I never thought of it that way!" We spoke further about some new professional opportunities she might have, and she left feeling more hopeful.

I am not suggesting that her emotional trauma was trivial or unwarranted. She did go through a great deal of discomfort and was still having a considerable amount of pain. That is not easy to live with. I've often wondered how I would react if faced with similar challenges. Nevertheless, the point is that she was grieving over the loss of a lifestyle that was not all that satisfying in the first place. She had not stopped to analyze her emotions, and this was leading to even more discomfort. Once she realized this, it freed her up to begin exploring new options, and she began an active search to determine what career would interest her.

I have seen a variation on this theme when a woman is going through a divorce. Many times she grieves not for the marriage as it was, but rather for the marriage as she wished it had been. If she can bring herself to analyze her situation truthfully, she frequently will realize that her needs were not being met and that the relationship was not all that satisfying.

This awareness is crucial if one wishes to avoid making the same mistakes over and over again. Too often, women will focus on the superficial failures in a marriage because it is too intimidating to tackle the real issues. Think about it. If your self-esteem depends solely on someone else's opinion, then a divorce is absolutely devastating because, in all but the rarest of circumstances, your soon-to-be ex no longer considers you the "ideal" woman.

Likewise, if you make others responsible for your happiness then you are setting yourself up for a fall. Since you cannot control another's behavior, it is risky to trust your happiness to someone else's judgment. Yet women do it all the time, sometimes multiple times with different partners. Understanding where your self-esteem impulses come from and understanding that you have a right to be happy is critical if you are going to break the cycle and achieve a satisfying life. You must be willing to analyze your reactions so that you can change behavior when you find something is not working out well. Otherwise, you will find yourself in the same unsatisfying situations again and again. And if you don't think that scenario plays havoc with your energy, think again!

## Anticipating Others' Reactions

There is another interesting phenomenon that will occur as you become more emotionally healthy and begin to set appropriate boundaries. Others in your sphere of influence—family, friends and colleagues—may well become upset with you. They may even get angry. I know this sounds odd, but here's why it happens. Whether you realize it or not, those around you are well aware of your self-esteem needs. It might not always be on a conscious level, but your family knows what strings to pull to make you respond in a certain way. So do the people you work and play with. Often they count on knowing those responses to get what they need or want. If you suddenly (at least it seems sudden) start thoughtfully evaluating their requests and realistically state what you can and cannot do, they are not going to like it. They will keep trying to pull those old strings that used to make you jump, and then become frustrated when they don't produce the desired response.

Here are some examples. The first involves a woman who was separated from her husband. He very confidently told a friend that she would never go through with a divorce because her "guilt would get her." He knew that would be a big issue for her because she belonged to a religion that did not recognize divorce. He believed it would be impossible for her to weather the disapproval from family and friends that was likely to follow her action. However, he did not realize that she had been working hard with a counselor to evaluate her marriage realistically and to deal more healthily with that constant need for approval. She eventually did finalize the divorce. On retelling, his confidence does seem pretty arrogant, but you must understand that he had years of data on which to base his assumption. She had changed; he just didn't notice, which may be a pertinent commentary on why the marriage failed!

The second example involves a woman's relationship with her parents. They were a close family and had always celebrated holidays together. Once she was married, they acknowledged the necessity for her to spend some holidays with her husband's family instead, but it seemed to her they always expressed their disappointment when that happened. She tried to ignore those comments because she knew it was unreasonable to expect her husband to forfeit all holiday celebrations with his family, and yet those holidays were often marred by feelings of guilt.

The incident that caught her attention and made her realize that she needed to change her response to the "guilt tugs" involved a trip with her husband to a meeting he was scheduled to attend. It was to be held in a lovely resort town, and he wanted her to go with him because he thought it would be a nice mini-vacation for them. Unfortunately, or fortunately since it led her to analyze her actions, this trip was over the Mother's Day weekend, which meant she would miss celebrating with her family.

She agonized over how she would tell her mother that she would be gone. She procrastinated for quite a while until it finally dawned on her that she was being silly. So she bit the bullet and made the call. Her mom was disappointed, but instead of the daughter's usual approach of apologizing and lamenting that she had "no choice but to go with her husband," the young woman simply remained pleasant and upbeat. In fact, she actually told her mom that she was looking forward to the trip. Her mom seemed a bit surprised that she was not apologetic, and after a few yanks on the guilt strings that did not elicit the desired response, she backed off and wished her a good time.

Does this anecdote remind you of any of the principles we've discussed in earlier chapters? It should. Remember, in Step 3, I urged you to challenge your assumptions, to put them through a reality filter so that you can be sure that you are accurately anticipating others' reactions. This young woman was correct in her assumption that her mother would be disappointed, but she completely overestimated the degree of disapproval that her trip would elicit. She was ready for a great deal of unpleasantness that simply did not occur.

It is a good lesson to learn as you begin to set boundaries. It is also the reason why I have stressed that you must follow the steps in sequence. Most assuredly, unless you are already in the habit of analyzing your responses, you will not have the tools to properly evaluate the reactions of others.

Of course, there will also be times when the response to your boundary setting is every bit as uncomfortable as you predicted. That's why it is important to have "done your homework." You need to be certain that the boundary you set is an appropriate one. You need to examine your motives to be confident that you are not acting out of anger, pettiness, guilt, or other less-than-healthy emotions. If so, then you need to rethink the process. You also need to evaluate and anticipate the effect the boundary will have on others, and factor that into your decision-making process. Remember, boundaries should be liberating, not limiting.

## Knowing When to Say When

If you are using a boundary to express discontent or to give someone an ultimatum, then that may not be healthy for you. There is an old rule espoused by consultants, "If it is emotionally satisfying, don't say it." To which I have added the corollary, "...and definitely, don't do it!" I try to always follow this adage. When I do, it has saved me embarrassment. When I don't, I end up with that uncomfortable feeling that tells me that my motivation was unhealthy. Then I have to go through the process of figuring out why I responded as I did and make amends if necessary. Believe me, it is easier and far less time-consuming to just follow the adage.

Boundaries are not a license to be selfish and self-serving. Notice that I use the word "appropriate" or "reasonable" frequently when I describe boundaries. You must be able to clearly delineate and understand your motivations if you wish to be successful at setting boundaries. Otherwise, you run the risk of simply being a tyrant—one who says, "It's my way or the highway." While that may be emotionally satisfying in the short run, it is ultimately unhealthy. Most important, it will not restore your energy.

On the other hand, if you have analyzed and determined that your motivation is healthy and your actions appropriate, then you simply have to go through with your plan, recognizing that you cannot control others' responses. A friend of mine is a recovering alcoholic. After he achieved sobriety, he found that he could no longer spend much time with his old friends. It wasn't that they were a bad influence because most of them were not heavy drinkers. Nevertheless, when he was with them, the temptation to drink was more that he could handle. In order to protect his tenuous sobriety, he had to limit his contact with them. Some understood, but others felt rejected. Some even became angry with him and told him they liked him better before he was sober. Their reactions naturally made him uncomfortable but did not deter him from the maintaining the boundaries that were necessary and appropriate for him.

His boundaries were a matter of survival, and it is easy to understand why they were necessary. However, focus your thoughts for a moment on situations that are not life-threatening, but which repeatedly end unsuccessfully. There is a saying in Alcoholics Anonymous that insanity is doing the same thing over and over again and expecting a different outcome. We often do this without even realizing how much it takes a toll on our energy.

Here's an example of a woman who was frustrated for years before she finally realized how foolish her actions were. She spoke with her mom regularly by phone. Often, she found that they would get into an argument over something inconsequential and would hang up exasperated with each other. The daughter always felt guilty after these exchanges and would usually call back to apologize even when she felt her mom had been the unreasonable one. It was a question of which was worse—the guilt she felt with her mom or the frustration she felt with capitulation.

This behavior continued for years until she finally realized it was unhealthy and energy draining. She resolved to be respectful toward her mom, to try to avoid the argument but, if it happened, to resist calling her mother back to smooth things over. It was difficult, but she knew she had to break the cycle. Interestingly, the first few times her mom called her back after a couple of hours to ask if "everything was okay" since she, too, had come to expect the follow-up call. The daughter remained pleasant, but purposely did not bring up the previous discussion. After a time, she found she no longer felt guilty, her mother did not expect an apology call, and their arguments actually became less frequent. They both learned a different way of interacting that was less time consuming and more satisfying.

Another friend of mine is a real take-charge person. She is a hard-driving executive and is respected for her problem-solving abilities. Her mother was getting older and would often speak with her daughter about whatever dilemma she was facing. Mom would ask the daughter what she thought she should do. The daughter would listen carefully and then offer different solutions for her mother to consider, but she invariably would become annoyed when her mom rejected them all explaining why each could not possibly work.

My friend finally realized her mother was not looking for solutions. What she really wanted to do was to express her frustration over the issues. Once the daughter became aware of this, she abandoned her irritation and adopted a new approach. Instead of telling her mom what to do, she simply listened to her concerns and offered encouraging words such as, "That is a difficult problem. I know you'll figure out the best way to handle it." She was not condescending, but respectful and interested. Above all, she resisted the urge to try to solve the problem. This worked well for both of them because now the daughter was really giving her mom what she needed and wanted.

This sounds like such a simple, obvious solution, but think about the steps involved. My friend had to analyze both her mother's reaction and her own. She had to accept that she would not change her mom's behavior, and she had to understand the source of her own frustration. Then she had to change her approach—and that is the key. As I've said over and over again, insight is not enough. You must use that insight to effect change, and that is precisely what she did. She set up a healthy boundary that was comfortable for both her and her mom.

## Start Small and Work Your Way Up

Boundaries do not have to involve earth-shattering issues. For example, one early boundary-setting success on my part came when I made sure each member of my family had enough underwear and socks to last a week. That way I only have to do laundry on the weekends, when it is easy to work in, instead of during the week when life is much more hectic.

My family knows that if they want something washed, they need to have it in before my weekly session or it will wait until the next week. Lauren now does her own laundry and has never been one of those college kids who bring it home as a gift for mom. When she lived at home, however, she would just do it herself if it was something she needed during the week. Understand that laundry is something that I like to do. I'm particular about it and count it as one of those nurturing things I do for my family. Therefore, before she left for college, I still retained this task, even though I taught her how to do it. But that was by choice, not obligation, and that makes all the difference.

I remember a funny anecdote with my mother-in-law involving the laundry and my fussiness about it. When Margaret first moved in with us after her diagnosis of lung cancer, she was still feeling quite well and wanted to help out around the house. She assumed (as many would!) that folding clothes would be something I would appreciate. However, after a few attempts with me hovering over her shoulder to be sure that she folded correctly, she suggested that maybe she would find some other way to help. I gratefully agreed, because in truth, it was driving me crazy. That's how particular I am about this task.

This issue resolved very easily for us because it was not clouded by other agendas. All she really wanted to do was help, and when she saw that that was not happening, she did not become angry, she simply looked for another avenue. Had she not approached it in this manner, I would have been faced with a decision. Either I would have needed to ask her not to the laundry, or I would have had

MARY ANN **BAUMAN, MD**

to accept gracefully what she did and how she did it. That's because it would not have been healthy for me to be repeatedly irritated and to expend energy on this issue. As it was, I was grateful for her perceptiveness, and we both laughed about the incident.

Another simple boundary I have established involves Christmas cards—I no longer send them. I found they were a major chore instead of a pleasure, and I did not need anything else to compete for my energy during the busy holiday season. As a consequence of that decision, I get fewer cards, but that is the price I pay and I accept it. My husband sometimes sends out cards when his spirit is moved to do so, and I do have a few out-of-town friends to whom I send a letter. I must confess, however, that it is sometimes Valentine's Day before I get them completed. You must also have patient, understanding friends if you adopt my approach!

Unlike me, my mom is an avid Christmas card sender. She writes notes on each one and delights in this correspondence. For her it is a pleasure and her gift to those who receive them. I admire that she takes the time to do this, but it just did not work for me. You see, boundaries do not always involve gut-wrenching situations. For me, Christmas cards did not represent a major issue. Sometimes, you simply need to use common sense to identify and eliminate some of your personal energy thieves.

## Personal and Professional Boundaries

You may have noticed that many of the examples I have cited involve the relationships we have with family members. That's because these are so often our most important and energy-draining interactions; thus providing great fodder for study and change. But the workplace is also awash with opportunities to set appropriate boundaries.

Sometimes, it may involve a simple situation such as designing a rotating schedule so that you are not the one who has to make the coffee every day. You will be amazed at how often a minor change will make a world of difference in how you feel. Remember, you use energy to nurture those little resentments that pepper your day. That's energy you cannot afford to waste.

Perhaps you are the person who "volunteers" on every occasion and later wonders how you are going to do it all. You then become irritated because people keep approaching you, when in fact you are the only one who can put a halt to your over-extension. It is not reasonable to fault those who do the asking. The inability to say "no" frequently is a manifestation of those sneaky self-esteem tentacles reaching out to bind you up once again. If you are constantly afraid that someone will think ill of you and your self-esteem is totally dependent on others' approval, then it is no wonder that you say "yes" far too frequently. It is difficult to set reasonable boundaries unless you have dealt with those well-meaning self-esteem demons.

I face the "just say no" scenario quite regularly in my professional life. I get many invitations to speak to groups, and it is something that I love to do. For me, there is nothing more gratifying and enjoyable than connecting with an audience. Not only is it fun, but it is a wonderful opportunity to educate people about a healthy lifestyle. It is also good for my career. Regardless of the benefits, I recognize that I have to carefully evaluate how much I can do. Otherwise, my mood and ultimately my energy will suffer. For example, I am fairly strict about limiting my evening engagements so that I don't encroach on family time. I also know that I need that downtime to recoup and rejuvenate, or even the things I enjoy will become a burden.

In our busy lives, there are so many demands on our time and energy that it is crucial for us to guard against those practices that do nothing but use up time and sap our energy. If you are thoughtful in this process, you will often be able to use these boundaries to forge healthier relationships with those you love and those you work with. Relationships based on proper assumptions with realistic boundaries are eminently satisfying.

# STEP 6: SET A BOUNDARY

This is the final step and the one that will most directly impact your energy balance. It's taken some effort to get here, but you're about to reap the rewards.

*You are ready to start setting appropriate boundaries in your everyday life. Start with a simple situation, perhaps one involving a family member or coworker. Anticipate the situation as you did in Step 5, analyze your feelings, and then inform the individual of the limits to your involvement.*

For example, if you are constantly ending the day by struggling with your children over homework, think the situation through and set reasonable boundaries. You could choose to tell your children that if they want you to check their homework, they must get it to you before 7 p.m. That gives you a chance to complete the task early enough so that you still have time in the evening for yourself.

I did this with Lauren during the years when she still needed my help, and it was quite successful. At first she balked because I was asking her to conform to my schedule, but I was firm, not angry, and she complied. Sometimes circumstances required that we alter the rule, but for the most part, we stuck to it. The added benefit was that she, too, had more free time in the evening. This simple boundary eliminated many irritating encounters.

*Be calm, reasonable, and pleasant, but not defensive. You might feel uncomfortable, but that's to be expected so play through it.*

I was not exaggerating when I said I had a hard time going out on my run that day I assumed my family disapproved. It wasn't easy to suppress those quick-to-surface feelings of guilt. Remember, you may or may not accurately predict the response to your request. If you've been thoughtful about the situation you have chosen, then stick to your plan. Ideally, you will be pleasantly surprised.

On the other hand, if the individual reacts in a negative way, you must listen to the objections and decide if they are compelling enough to warrant a change in your boundary request. Take care to examine the objections accurately. If you are not careful, you will draw on those firmly entrenched approval tendencies, and you will let that need dictate your actions. Sometimes you have to be willing to accept that something that may be right for you may irritate others.

It is best initially to choose situations that are low-risk and have a likely chance of success. That way you can gain some experience and confidence before you tackle some of the more important boundaries you may need to establish. Be creative in finding those circumstances that will simplify your life and in devising ways to limit them. Setting appropriate boundaries in small, seemingly inconsequential situations will help you to approach the larger issues with more confidence.

Sometimes we have a tendency to minimize our successes with disparaging comments such as, "That was such a little thing so it really doesn't matter." Avoid this pitfall; learn to accept success gracefully. Recognize what you did to accomplish it so you can build on those positive experiences. Similarly, if you met with resistance to your boundary, don't become discouraged. Learn from the experience and approach similar situations differently the next time. Above all, do not berate yourself. Not only is that nonproductive, it is counter-productive—it defeats the purpose.

This step will not work if you have not made the other five a part of your routine. That's because it presupposes that you have already accepted the mind-body influence in your daily life, that you are able to analyze your reactions to your day-to-day encounters, and that you recognize when your self-esteem-driven need for approval threatens your energy reserves. It assumes that you are ready to change your behavior—and that pays great dividends.

# CHAPTER 7

# THE FINALE—AND THE "MISSING" PIECES

In the past six chapters we have covered a lot of material, but there are some subject areas I have deliberately avoided or treated very briefly. There were reasons for each of these decisions, and we'll discuss a few of them in a moment.

Before we talk about what we *haven't* covered, however, let's talk about what we *have* covered. My undergraduate education was in engineering, and we were always taught to break a problem into its component pieces before you tackle solutions, and that is just what we have done as we launched you on the journey to maximize your energy. We began this whole process by introducing the concept that our self-esteem needs are heavily responsible for our energy crisis. We then outlined a two-phased approach to begin changing this pattern.

Take a moment to review the two phases and the six steps they contain. Then we'll address what's missing and why.

# PHASE ONE

## ANALYZING THE RELATIONSHIPS IN YOUR LIFE

### Step 1: Identify.

At some time during your day, think about one encounter you had during the previous 24 hours. Decide if that interaction made you happy or sad, satisfied or resentful, comfortable or uneasy. You have a whole range of reactions from which to choose. As the days go by, try to recall a mix of both positive and negative experiences.

Be careful not to overanalyze the encounter. You will be tempted to focus on negative encounters so that's why it is critical that you choose some situations where the outcome was positive. There are many times during each day that you do things well. Now is the time to remember them. Do this daily until it becomes a regular part of your life. It must become a habit and the only way that will happen is by repetition.

## Step 2: Evaluate.

Once you feel comfortable with the identification process you can begin to evaluate your daily encounters. Remember to choose a new encounter each day.

Now, not only do you decide how the encounter made you feel afterward, but also consider how you felt just prior to the episode. Were you happy? Angry? Rushed? Annoyed? Tired? Hungry? Scared? You are trying to determine your emotional state at the time because this almost always influences the choices you make. Poor choices lead to dissatisfaction and eventually overextension as you try to compensate.

## Step 3: Challenge.

Once you can routinely identify your emotions at the time of an incident, you are ready to start challenging your assumptions. Think for a moment about what you thought would happen in the encounter before it occurred. Then compare it with what actually did happen. In this way, you are testing the validity of your assumptions, and those assumptions often determine how you will respond to a situation.

To summarize the analysis steps: First, you identify how you feel after an encounter. Next, you evaluate how you felt prior to the episode. And finally, you challenge the accuracy of your assumptions. Now it's time to begin to change your behavior.

## PHASE TWO

### CHANGING THE WAY YOU HANDLE RELATIONSHIPS

#### Step 4: Break down the barriers.

Some barriers are obvious, but others are much more cleverly hidden. In this step you will take a double-pronged approach. You will break down the barriers to exercise while at the same time acknowledging and attacking some of the other barriers that can affect your energy. It is important to work on both. Exercise is critical to the restoration of your energy so begin by making exercise your priority. If you like the idea of the reward system to induce you to exercise, then concentrate on identifying that reward. Remember to choose a reward that is readily available, since you will be enjoying it multiple times a week.

Once again, it's important to keep it simple. Force yourself to get your body moving three to four times a week, rain or shine, stressed or relaxed, time or no time. Reject any barriers in your path but don't be critical. If you couldn't do as much as you had planned, vow to do

MARY ANN **BAUMAN, MD**

better the next time, be happy with what you did, and move on.

Set reasonable expectations. Your goal is to be successful so don't sabotage that.

As we've discussed, though, there are many other barriers that, if allowed to remain in place, will siphon off your energy. You must identify those and break them down one by one. Start with an easy one and find a way to make it work. Be careful to choose barriers that you do, in fact, control. When you select something that is beyond your scope of influence, you are setting yourself up for failure. Remember that all barriers are not monumental so you want to actively look for the small ones that cause annoyances, irritation, and delays in your day. Those, added up, will take a cumulative toll on your energy reserves.

It's always advisable to have some successes under your belt before you tackle some of the most difficult barriers, usually those that involve the important people in your life. Don't rush it. Remember, this step is part of a plan that all fits together and is designed to help you to gradually change the way you approach your life situations.

### Step 5: Explore and experiment.

What if you could go back and relive this day's encounter? If the incident was negative, is there anything you could have done differently to elicit a more positive outcome? If it was positive, can you pinpoint why? What action or reaction on your part elicited the response? Think of how often a negative encounter happened because you were stressed, angry, or tired. The point is that had you handled the initial actions differently, the outcome might have been quite different.

Be good to yourself, though. You must also recognize those times when you handled a situation well and were rewarded with a pleasant response. Visualize how easily an encounter could have turned sour if you hadn't demonstrated the wisdom and foresight to handle it smoothly.

Now try new approaches. Start experimenting with different ways to handle situations. Choose an upcoming interaction. Try to set the scene, analyze the factors that will influence you, and visualize possible outcomes. Then use the healthy behaviors that you've previously identified to encourage a positive result. If your first plan doesn't work, pick another encounter with the same person and go back to the drawing board. Alternatively, take on an upcoming meeting with another individual and try again. Through trial and error, you can be successful. You build self-esteem one encounter at a time.

Be sure to explore and experiment with rewards as well. Take the time to figure out what gives you pleasure. Find your rewards and then indulge on a regular basis. You must do something for yourself at least once a week so make certain that some of your rewards are realistic and conducive to that.

Remember the cautions that accompany this step: First, be honest with yourself as you do the exploration and experimentation. After all, you are the only person in the audience. You are not trying to impress anyone else. Second, don't overestimate your own role. You cannot always control the outcome of a situation. One of the most valuable skills we can learn is to willingly take responsibility for our own behavior, but not the behavior of others, good or bad. The challenge is learning to recognize what is yours to change. It becomes easier when you learn to focus objectively on your performance. That will happen when your self-esteem is no longer at risk whenever someone hints at disapproval or when you even think they are hinting at disapproval.

Once again, you must keep up this process until it becomes second nature to you. Continue to evaluate your encounters to see if they could have or should have been handled differently, and acknowledge those that go well.

### Step 6: Set a boundary.

You are now ready to begin setting appropriate boundaries in your everyday life. Start with a simple situation. Anticipate the situation as you did in Step 4, analyze your feelings, and then inform the individual of the limits to your involvement. Be calm, reasonable, and pleasant, but not defensive. You might feel uncomfortable, but that's to be expected so play through it. If you've been thoughtful about the situation you have chosen, then stick to your plan. Remember, you may or may not accurately predict the response to your request.

On the other hand, if the individual reacts in a negative way, you must listen to the objections and decide if they are compelling enough to warrant a change in your boundary request. Take care to examine the objections accurately but realize that sometimes you have to be willing to accept that a decision that is right for you may irritate others.

Initially, choose situations that are low-risk and have a likely chance of success so that you can gain some experience and confidence before you tackle some of the more important boundaries you may need to establish. All boundaries do not have to be earth shattering. Sometimes, you simply need to use common sense to identify and eliminate some of your personal energy thieves. Be creative.

Take care not to minimize your successes. Accept them gracefully and recognize what you did to accomplish them so you can build on those positive experiences. Similarly, if you met with resistance to your boundary, don't become discouraged. Learn from the experience and approach similar situations differently the next time. Above all, do not berate

MARY ANN **BAUMAN, MD**

yourself. Not only is that nonproductive, it is counterproductive—it defeats the purpose.

## A Continuing Journey

So there you have them. Six steps, not terribly difficult, not terribly time consuming, requiring only that you follow them in order and consistently. I know you can be successful, if you are willing make the commitment. As I asked in my introduction, what will you have to lose except that exhausted feeling at the end of your day?

They do work. They've worked for me and for many of my patients, but you must commit yourself to establishing healthy self-esteem habits. You must evaluate your behavior on an ongoing basis so that you will learn to recognize when you slip back into your "people-pleasing" mode. That is the way to avoid making commitments that stretch you beyond your limits and rob you of energy. Sometimes it is impossible to avoid such commitments, of course, but you may be surprised at how seldom this really occurs. In the vast majority of cases, you can control the situation if you are willing to identify and set boundaries.

This is an ongoing process. It is not something that you accomplish once and then consider finished. The demands you face are not single, one-time events. They change through the days, months, and years with fresh demands on your time and energy cropping up frequently. Just when you think you've eliminated your energy thieves, new ones replace the old. But, if you are diligently working the steps, you'll quickly become aware of them, and you won't need to become totally exhausted, angry, and frustrated before you take corrective action.

Awhile ago, I found myself in this situation. Changes occurred in our marketplace that forced a business change in my medical practice. I'm just like most other people—I do not readily and enthusiastically embrace change, especially when dictated by someone else! So predictably, I'd been experiencing some stress as our group figured out how to respond.

What's more, during this same time period, my annual series of seminars to high school students began, obligating me to spend a fair amount of time out of the office. That always lengthens my day, as I have to take care of my patients' needs either early in the morning or late in the afternoon. Also, I still had my regularly scheduled 7 a.m. meetings during the week. Therefore, I continued to start early even though I was working later than usual during this time. Since I was getting home later, I was also going to bed later in order to still have my much-needed downtime. And then, because I was stressed, I found myself waking up even before my alarm rang. Get the picture? I was feeling more stressed, working later, and getting less sleep. For me, that is a recipe for exhaustion because I am a person who needs my sleep.

Now even though I have been working these steps for years, it still took me a couple of months and a forgotten speaking engagement! to realize that I had to make some changes. Here's what I did. First, I changed my patient schedule so that I see patients in the morning instead of the afternoon. I'm fresher then and more efficient. Second, I started taking my shower and washing my hair in the evening instead of in the morning. That allowed me an extra half hour of sleep each day. Third, I made it a point to not start watching the 10 p.m. newscast. Whenever I started the news program, I always seemed to stay up until it finished. To avoid this, I left to prepare for bed before it began. That added another half hour of sleep. Finally, I cleared my schedule of any engagements that were not crucial. This meant not attending the charity auction of an organization for which I am a board member, but I decided I needed the time at home to just relax. I called the event organizers and honestly told them why I would not attend. They were most gracious and even suggested the name of a couple that could attend instead of my husband and me.

None of these adjustments were earth shattering, but they worked. I was able to increase the number of patients in my practice, get an extra hour of sleep each night, and the auction went on without me with great success. I began to sleep better, no more of those early morning wake-ups, and the tired, stressed feeling disappeared.

Look at the process that led me to these changes, and notice how it reflects the six steps we just reviewed: First, I analyzed my reactions to determine why I was feeling so stressed (Step 1). I tried to anticipate how I would feel if I did go to the auction (Step 2). I examined my assumptions to be sure that the changes I thought I needed in my practice were really necessary (Step 3). I evaluated the barriers to getting enough sleep (Step 4), and then I experimented with new approaches on several different fronts (Step 5). Finally, I set reasonable boundaries for my disposable time (Step 6) and made those who needed to know aware of my decision.

Notice, too, what I did not do. I did not berate myself for taking too long to realize why I was stressed. I did not blame others (well, maybe a little!) for the situation that led to the need for changes in my practice. I did not make up an excuse to the auction organizers about why I would not attend. Those are all unhelpful reactions and will not result in constructive problem solving. Negative emotions simply eat up your energy. You must guard against them.

Remember, if you tend to be pessimistic, your first task is always to find the positive in any situation, no matter how slight or inconsequen-

MARY ANN **BAUMAN, MD**

tial that positive may be. You must recognize that small changes can pay big dividends, and you have to give yourself the credit you deserve when you do start to make changes. There is a well-deserved sense of accomplishment that comes from being proactive. Even if your first change is not successful, it will serve as a catalyst for the next one.

A colleague who does quite a number of research studies once told me that when he first began, he had the hardest time trying to find a research idea. However, once he finished the first study, the ideas came so fast that he did not have enough time to pursue them all. The same is true of the process we've been exploring. Once you have mastered the analysis phase and have had some success with boundary setting, you will find yourself eager to continue the process. Trust me; it is a powerful feeling when you begin to attack the energy thieves in your life.

On the other hand, don't expect that your people-pleasing tendencies will simply disappear. The self-esteem-driven, need-for-approval tendencies will crop up periodically. The difference, however, is that you will now recognize them for what they are, understand where they come from, and not waste much precious energy trying to appease them. Over time, these episodes will happen less frequently.

## What We Haven't Discussed

Now as promised, a few comments about what I deliberately did *not* address in this book. First, let's talk about something that is not required for this plan to be successful. You may have noticed that I have not insisted that you keep a journal for any of these six steps. Writing down experiences doesn't work for everyone, including me. If you told me that I had to write about each encounter in order to achieve mind-body balance and maximize my energy, I would give up immediately. Journaling just does not fit into my lifestyle. It would just be another task to add to my busy schedule.

I've designed these steps to be done while you are pursuing your daily activities, not in addition to them. However, if you find that recording experiences helps you to focus and follow your progress, then by all means write them down. Find the technique that works for you. This is your journey, and there is no set timetable. You'll know it's working when you feel the resurgence of your energy and find joy in your life.

Another point I have deliberately omitted relates to how women and men achieve self-esteem. I began with the premise that women and men develop self-esteem in different ways. You may wonder why I did not challenge that assumption or why I did not suggest that women become more task-oriented and less driven by relationships.

In fact, I believe that women do complete multiple tasks every day, and it is important that we recognize and respect our accomplishments. However, it is our responses to the relationships in our lives that often deplete our energy reserves. Remember when I was disappointed that driving my daughter to school was a stressful time for both of us? When I spoke about it with my husband, I learned that on those occasions when he did the drive, he and Lauren hardly spoke at all. And it didn't matter to him; he was most interested in getting her to school on time.

Both of us completed the task, but just completing the task was not what was most important to me. I wanted to use the time for bonding, and when that didn't happen, it affected the rest of my day. It wasn't the task that bothered me; I finished that easily. *It was the relationship.*

I once read an interesting anecdote about the invention of the vacuum cleaner. It was designed to free women from the drudgery of cleaning their carpets and rugs. What actually happened, however, was quite the opposite: Instead of beating their rugs once a week, women began vacuuming their floors every day. This wonderful timesaver actually added to the household workload! So it is with our self-esteem. If we simply focus on accomplishing more tasks without paying attention to how our relationships fit into the equation, we will add to both our physical and emotional workloads, and we will not be happy.

In the introduction of this book, I invited you to begin a journey with me. I deliberately chose this word because I truly believe that we are on a journey and one of our most challenging tasks on that journey is to figure out why we do what we do. We do have the ability to change our behavior, but we must first recognize when it is unhealthy, unsatisfying, or both. We must also learn to celebrate our achievements. Too often, we are unwilling or unable to acknowledge those things we do well.

The self-esteem issues we have delineated are real, and they impact our lives every single day. Mind-body balance will bring joy to your life, and the wonderful byproduct of this is abundant energy. I wish you health, wellness, and success on your journey. Be good to yourself.

# REFERENCES

Atkinson H, 1985. *Women and fatigue*. New York: Putnam.

Berk LS, Tan SA, Fry WF. 1989. Neuroendocrine and stress hormone changes during mirthful laughter. *The American Journal of the Medical Sciences* 298(6):390–96.

Cousins N.1979. *Anatomy of an illness as perceived by the patient: reflections on healing and regeneration*. New York: Norton.

Frankel MT. 1991. Does father know best? Mothers and fathers teaching their preschool sons and daughters. Abstract: March.

Jemmott JB 3rd, Magloire K. 1988. Academic stress, social support, and secretory immunoglobulin A. *Journal of Personality and Social Psychology* 55(5):803–10.

Kubzansky LD, Sparrow D, Vokonas P. 2001. Is the glass half empty or half full? A prospective study of optimism and coronary heart disease in the normative aging study. *Psychosomatic Medicine* 63(6):910–16.

Lee PCL, Jawad MSM, Hull JD, West WHL, et al. 2005. The antitussive effect of placebo treatment on cough associated with acute upper respiratory infection. *Psychosomatic Medicine* 67(2):314–17.

Martikainen P, Valkonen T. 1998. Do education and income buffer the effects of death of spouse on mortality? *Epidemiology* 9(5):530–4.

Neifert MR, Price A, Dana N. 1986. *Dr Mom: a guide to baby and child care.* New York: Putnam.

Peterson C, Vaillant GE, Seligman MEP. 1988. Pessimistic explanatory style is a risk factor for physical illness: a thirty-five year longitudinal study. *Journal of Personality and Social Psychology* 55(1):23–7.

Rider MS, Achterberg J, Lawlis GF, Goven A, et al. 1990. Effect of immune system imagery on secretory IgA. *Biofeedback & Self Regulation* 15(4):317–33.

Wolf S. 1950. Effects of suggestion and conditioning on the action of chemical agents in human subjects: the pharmacology of placebos. *Journal of Clinical Investigation* 29:100–9.

Contact Dr. Mary Ann Bauman at
www.maryannbaumanMD.com

or order more copies of this book at:

TATE PUBLISHING, LLC

127 East Trade Center Terrace
Mustang, Oklahoma 73064

(888) 361 - 9473

TATE PUBLISHING, LLC
www.tatepublishing.com